FOR
WANT
OF A
CHILD

FOR WANT OF A CHILD

A Psychologist and His Wife Explore the Emotional Effects and Challenges of Infertility

James McGuirk
and
Mary Elizabeth McGuirk

Foreword by William Van Ornum

Continuum | New York

1991

The Continuum Publishing Company
370 Lexington Avenue
New York, NY 10017

Printed in the United States of America

Library of Congress Cataloging-in-Publication Data

McGuirk, James.
    For want of a child : a psychologist and his wife explore the
emotional effects and challenges of infertility / James McGuirk and
Mary Elizabeth McGuirk ; foreword by William Van Ornum.
        p.   cm.
    Includes bibliographical references.
    ISBN 0-8264-0493-6
    1. Infertility—Psychological aspects.   I. McGuirk, Mary
Elizabeth.   II. Title.   III. Series.
RC889.M377   1991
155.9'16—dc20

                                                                    90–45652
                                                                    CIP

To Sean

Contents

Foreword

Infertility, as the authors point out, is an emotional syndrome as well as a medical condition that affects many others beyond the couple themselves, especially the grandparents and other extended family members. What is unique about this book is that this difficult problem is discussed by a practicing psychologist and his wife who have themselves struggled with infertility. They have written a book that has the "ring of authenticity" about what is a challenging and troubling problem for many.

Jim and Beth McGuirk start by talking about their hope for having children and the sadness they faced with the realization that they were not able to conceive. Their book becomes a shared journey of what they learned as they worked together to understand the condition. Happily, their journey ends with the adoption of their son.

This book will be helpful to anyone struggling with infertility or for family, friends, or other helpers who are working with such persons. And, in our society, there may be more couples like this than most of us realize. As the McGuirks point out, "for fifteen to twenty percent of couples, the expectations are not fulfilled and for many, their dreams are crushed. They are diagnosed infertile." This book is written to help these couples look at the options available to them. Medical, financial, and emotional issues are discussed in a comprehensive and compassionate manner. Whereas the biological aspects are summarized, the main focus of the book is on the emotional impact on the person and the couple. Readers will also find many kinds of practical information, such as a description of the different medical specialists they might encounter.

Issues of separation and loss are powerful and can be difficult to understand intellectually, especially regarding infertility, miscarriage, and stillbirth and the McGuirks point out how grieving can be difficult because there may not be cultural rituals for these types of loss.

There is an awareness of the sadness that may be present, but a theme of hopefulness runs through the book. There are many things that couples can do themselves and the McGuirks encourage them to "take charge of treatment." Although infertility is a condition that can add stress to a marriage, the McGuirks report that "research also indicates that struggling with infertility can result in strong marital bonds." They provide practical communication strategies that will be helpful to couples. In addition, they speak of the many aspects related to resolving infertility, and readers will be touched by the manner in which their struggle ended happily.

For Want of a Child is not only a practical book, it is a book that will touch the hearts of couples, their family and friends, and those who help them. The personal and professional experiences of the McGuirks will inspire all who read this book.

William Van Ornum, Ph.D.
Marist College
Poughkeepsie, New York

For Want of a Child

Acknowledgments

Major projects are never completed without the assistance and support of many people. This project was no different. We learned early on that we would need considerable help if the book was to provide the type of information that we wanted and was to be presented in a way that would convey the emotional message that was the focus of this book.

We would like to start by giving heartfelt thanks to those couples and individuals who agreed to be interviewed for this book. Because we promised anonymity, we cannot thank each person by name. Friends, co-workers, and strangers agreed to share their most personal thoughts with us. Without them, our book would not have the depth of feeling that we believe is critical to making the content real.

We also want to thank our family for the support they provided as we worked on this book. As was the case through our struggle with infertility, our family was encouraging and supportive at all times. We want to give a special thanks to our parents, Frances and Edward Adams, and Rosemary and Joseph McGuirk. As the deadline grew nearer and the pressure to complete the book increased, they agreed to baby-sit for our son. We know it was "a tough job that somebody had to do."

We also received much support and encouragement from our friends. Whether at home or at work, our friends were understanding and patient as we were confronting our difficult feelings. With the book, they always showed an interest in the project and a willingness to help. At the Astor Home for Children, David Crenshaw and Laura Worth provided boundless support as they shared their struggles with completing books that are also part of this series. Special appreciation is given to Teresa Brettschneider, the librarian at the Astor Home, who did the initial computer search and hunted for the books and articles we needed for our information. We want to thank Amy Pass. She cared for our son while we worked to complete this project. We also want to thank Dr. William Van Ornum for his encouragement through the process. Just as we were getting discouraged, he was able to give us a lift and help us to the next stage of the project.

Finally, we cannot finish without acknowledging the many infertile couples who simply by their presence made our suffering more bearable. As we eventually realized, and we hope readers learn from this work, life's challenges seem easier when you know you are not alone.

Introduction

When we were first married, we shared an assumption held by most married couples that we could have children whenever we wanted. For the first five years of our marriage, one of our worst unspoken fears was that we would give birth to a child before we were ready. We went to considerable trouble to prevent conception. Eventually, like many married couples, we took on the additional stress of planning and attempting to agree as a couple that we were finally ready for children. Thus, we proceeded with what we assumed would be an easy and even enjoyable process of attempting to become pregnant.

It did not take us long to realize that the process would not be as exciting as we had anticipated. Soon we discovered it would not be easy. It took much longer for us to realize having children would be stressful for us. After a year, we learned we had joined a growing number of couples that are diagnosed as infertile. This simple diagnosis would change our feelings about ourselves, would challenge us as individuals and as a couple, and would stress us to points that we previously thought we would never be able to handle. We suffered considerably with our simple diagnosis, but we also grew.

Infertility is a problem couples have struggled with since the beginning of time. However, as a growing number of baby boomers move into child-bearing years, albeit later in life compared to previous generations, infertility has become more publicized as a problem. Current estimates suggest that 10,000,000 people a year experience infertility. Recent incident estimates indicate that from 15 to 20 percent of couples will have to deal with infertility during their lifetimes. More specifically, couples who put off having children until relatively later in life have a greater risk of being infertile. Twenty-five percent of couples in

15

their thirties will have difficulty having children as compared to 1 percent of teenage couples.

Infertility is not a problem that limits its effect to the infertile couple. Also affected are a large number of frustrated grandparents-to-be, siblings, and friends. They are aware of the problems, but for the most part do not understand the range of emotions the couple is experiencing. For us, many supposed happy occasions have turned sour when another couple shares their "good news," that they will soon be parents. Instead of the excitement expected at such announcements, the parents-to-be are met with anger, sadness, or at best, contained feelings not fully shared.

Infertility is as much an emotional syndrome as it is a medical condition. The longer a couple struggles with the problem, the more likely they are to face a series of emotional challenges that puts even the best of marriages at risk. People deal with the stress of infertility as they would with any other stressor. The better the coping mechanism, the more successful the couple will be in dealing with the challenge.

Experience suggests that gaining knowledge about infertility and its causes enhances couples' coping abilities. When couples look to counselors, clergy, and other helping professionals for support and assistance, they may be looking for answers to basic questions, guidelines about what direction to follow in their search for an answer, or support and understanding for what seems to be overwhelming emotions. Helpers who understand the dynamics of infertility are better prepared to provide the range of assistance often required.

We discuss the medical and emotional dynamics of infertility. We expect that the book will be helpful to several groups of readers. One group is the wide range of professionals who may have contact with infertile couples. This group includes psychologists, social workers, counselors, nurses and clergy who are in a position to work with couples who are infertile. For the most part, helping professionals do not understand the impact of infertility on couples' lives. Even physicians who are well schooled in the medical aspects of infertility may not be as aware as they should be of the psychological experience.

We also hope that infertile couples will benefit from the book. The book is a shared journey. We describe the emotions couples have experienced or can expect to experience as they face the problem. We provide suggestions that attempt to alleviate anxiety and pain, and to improve coping abilities.

Finally, the book may provide assistance to friends and relatives of the infertile. Often, friends and relatives want to help, but do not know how. If they have some understanding of the emotions couples are experiencing, they will be better able to show their concern for the couples' dilemma. We want those people who read this book to have a better understanding of the emotions that boil up in those couples faced with infertility and to gain some ideas about how to help infertile couples.

Authors' Note

The identities of the individuals in the case studies of this book have been carefully disguised in accordance with professional standards of confidentiality and in keeping with their rights to privileged communication with the authors.

1

A Woman's Perspective

Yet woman will be saved through bearing children
1 Timothy 2:15

I WAS VERY EXCITED when we decided to start our family. Although Jim was in graduate school, I figured we could handle having a baby too. I think my anxiety to get going overshadowed the reality of the situation. As I look back, I think it would have been difficult having a child at that time, financially and emotionally. But not as difficult as what was to follow.

After about four or five months of trying to conceive I began to get worried. I knew it had taken my mother several years to have a baby and I was afraid it was going to be the same way for me.

We agreed to wait before talking to my gynecologist, and started the basal body temperature (BBT) charts on our own. Despite our decision to try on our own for a while, I couldn't wait for long and made an appointment after only eight months. My doctor's response was that I was only twenty-six-years old, we had not been trying for a full year, and she did not want to start testing until that time. She gave us a book to read about fertility and conception, and I sweated out the last months until testing would begin.

I was anxious to get started with the tests because I thought for sure my gynecologist would find the reason for our problem and take care of it.

We began with some basic blood tests and the postcoital test. I didn't mind the postcoital at all. I knew I was going to do

21

whatever I had to, and I looked at it all from a clinical viewpoint. When the postcoital was negative, I scheduled the hysterosalpingogram. I was not warned about how painful the procedure would be and that is when I first became very angry that I had to go through all this. Even though they didn't find anything wrong, the test itself must have done something because I became pregnant two months later.

We were very happy, as were our family and friends. This happened around the Christmas holidays, so there were additional baby gifts under the tree. Just after Christmas everything came crashing down. I started to have some spotting, but initially refused to believe that anything was wrong. However, as the day went on, it continued. My fear about having a miscarriage was confirmed and we were on our way to the hospital.

I had to stay overnight in the hospital. They put me in a private room, but I was evidently near the labor and delivery rooms because I could hear women screaming in pain all night. I was so angry that this was happening to me, to us. I felt so empty. I couldn't stop crying.

I had clung to a little bit of hope through the night that everything might be all right. It wasn't. The next morning the doctor told me, in a very unsympathetic manner, that my pregnancy test was negative and that I would have to have a D & C.

Even though I was sad, I kept telling myself that miscarriages are very common and that I'll soon be pregnant again. I was. This time it was different. I had gone through a full three months with no problems, but the ultrasound revealed a blighted ovum. Another D & C, another letdown.

I did conceive again after only a few months. I felt for sure this time that everything would be all right. I had filled my quota for miscarriages. This pregnancy was not meant to be either. I couldn't believe it had happened again.

My sister-in-law had gotten pregnant around the time of my second pregnancy. After I miscarried, it was very hard for me to accept her pregnancy. I was very angry and jealous that her pregnancy was allowed to continue. I tried to avoid her whenever I could. It didn't seem fair. When my niece was born it was hard for me to accept her at first. When I found out I was pregnant again it became much easier.

During all the miscarriages Jim was very supportive. I don't remember talking a great deal about the details of the events or even about our feelings; it was just something we both understood. I know he was as disappointed as I was, but he let me do all the crying.

Most everyone seemed sympathetic and I don't really remember any comments that made me angry or upset. But what did bother me were the people who didn't say anything to us about the miscarriages. Maybe they thought they were being kind by not mentioning them. Maybe because the miscarriages happened so early in the pregnancies they didn't really think that the babies were real to us. The emotions were all too real.

After the last miscarriage we went through more testing. They found several problems related to miscarrying and I went through several treatments, including one that was still somewhat experimental. I still hadn't given up and I was sure that something was going to work. But that wasn't going to happen, and the months turned into years.

During those years of testing and treatment I became very moody, jealous, angry, and bitter. I was angry that I had to suffer through all the probing, tests, surgery, side affects of medication, continuous visits to the doctor's office and the expense and emotional upheaval. One surgical procedure had to be canceled at the last minute after I had spent weeks emotionally preparing for it. I found myself yelling at the doctor and staff, something I thought I never would do.

News of friends' and relatives' pregnancies became increasingly hard to deal with. At the time, I never felt I was truly happy for them, even though I wanted to be. I found myself avoiding them more and dreading the baby-shower invitations. Some I did attend out of obligation, but they were usually difficult to get through.

Christmas also seemed to be more depressing as the years went on. We still continued to decorate and put up a tree, even though our hearts weren't in it. I tried to keep everything light because I felt I had to help Jim get through it. We did actually consider going away this last Christmas if we didn't have a baby by then. But by Christmas time we were lucky to have our son with whom to share the holiday.

We had talked about adoption several years earlier, but I was not ready to go through with it. I felt, at that time, that by adopting I was giving up and admitting failure. I was more consumed with the idea of getting pregnant than by rearing a child. As our friends and relatives began to have children, naturally and by adoption, I realized that what I really wanted was a baby. By now I understood that having a child didn't have to mean that I would get pregnant.

We now have a beautiful son that came into our family by adoption. As I go about my daily routine I look at him and wonder what we ever did without him. I can't imagine him in another family. He is truly ours.

The pain of my infertility diminishes a little more each day. My son has done that for me. Although I would still like to experience pregnancy, it doesn't matter as much to me now as it once did. I am enjoying every day so much more now. Even though my infertility is not cured, and every once in a while a jealous pang pops up when I see a pregnant woman, I look at my son's smiling face and say, "This is what it's all about."

T hroughout the ages, there has been an interdependency between women's sense of self and the ability to reproduce. One wonders if God realized that when He commanded Adam and Eve to be fruitful and multiply, women would bear the brunt of that burden.

Fertility has been valued in all cultures since the beginning of time. During the Victorian age, the ability to reproduce became the core of femininity and most closely related to women's self-identity. Motherhood was the path to fulfillment for Victorian-age women.[1] Women who were infertile were viewed by society as less feminine and less complete.

The relationship between femininity and fertility developed further after World War II. Freudian psychology taught that women's desire to have children was a psychic substitute for their desire to have a penis. According to Freud, women's desire to bear children was essential to their mental health. Thus, little girls were taught that their goal in life would be to bear children and rear a family.[2]

Freud's views were widely accepted and they supported the gender-based role differentiation that was common through much of the twentieth century. In the fifties, as the birthrate in the United States increased dramatically, motherhood continued to be the main role for the majority of women. In 1962, a Gallup poll showed that 90 percent of women called childbirth the most satisfying moment in their lives.[3] In our present age, women have found other ways, in addition to reproduction and motherhood, to feel good about themselves. Yet the ability to bear children remains a prominent part of many women's self-identity.

> "She had movie star parents, grew up in Hollywood and became a star in her own right. But Jamie Lee Curtis longed for something more: 'I wanted a child' "[4]

The Woman's Struggle with Others

We live in a society where a person's value as a member of our society is judged by the ability to be productive. For infertile women, their inability to reproduce makes them feel less valued and estranged from the fertile world. Feelings associated with infertility often result in women becoming isolated.

Infertility is often referred to as an invisible problem. However, the absence of children is visible to others, or so it seems to the infertile. Involuntary childlessness is considered a social condition.[5] Women who are infertile believe that they have been unfairly singled out; that they are the only ones without children. As more and more friends of infertile women have children, this belief soon turns to reality.

Although men struggle with similar issues, the social pressure seems to weigh more heavily on women. The type of pressure has a broad range. In extreme situations, some in-laws have been known to ask their daughter-in-law to divorce their son so he could marry a fertile woman.

The sense of difference between the fertile and infertile is reinforced when women feel they must put on a smiling facade to discuss their childlessness. Most infertile women resent questions about their plans for starting a family. Some will lie, stating that they choose not to have children. Others explain that they are simply not ready, for financial or career reasons. As one woman says, "It makes it easy for me to get out of situations." Yet, these answers don't tell the whole story because the hurt remains. Sometimes the hurt turns to anger.

> "Do you have any children yet?" or "Where are your kids?" or something like that. . . . At first—it's changed over time—I kind of say, no, we're trying and that's how I'd leave it. And then I'd say to myself, the nerve that they should be asking me! Why do people ask such personal questions? And then . . . some people come out and they'll say, "Well, why not? When are you going to?" I mean they push the subject. And then one time, someone was really pushing me and . . . asking me one question after another and finally I just turned to her and I said, "Because I can't have any children and we're trying to do something about it now. Just leave me alone." And I walked off. I was kind of rude but she pushed me to the limit.[6]

Women who are infertile become outraged when they think that others seem to have babies so easily or undeservingly. The apparent inconsistencies between the effort and the reward of a child are not easily understood. Many infertile women feel they are entitled to be angry and become upset at others' pregnancies. However, when people around them feel uncomfortable with the anger and try to minimize the feelings, or suggest the women should not get so upset, the situation can escalate. Infertile women rightfully believe, "Nobody has the right to tell me how I'm supposed to feel."

Comments made by others, usually without thinking, can be hurtful because they diminish the seriousness of the situation. Infertile women learn to cope with them in a way that allows them to deal with the pain experienced. If the cause for the infertility is known, some women find it helpful to talk about it. If they can explain in medical terms exactly what is wrong, unwarranted comments may be avoided. However, attempts to handle these types of questions with honesty often result in comments such as "Just relax" or "Adopt and you'll get pregnant." As a result, it becomes easier to avoid others rather than deal with these awkward situations.

Counselors, clergy, and other helpers can be very supportive to infertile women. So many people discount or minimize infertile women's anger and hurt. As a result, many women who are infertile do not realize that the feelings are a normal part of their infertility. Counselors can be helpful by listening to and accepting the feelings communicated. Thus, the women can be assisted in understanding that their feelings are as much a part of infertility as are the physical problems.

Counselors, clergy, and other helpers can also assist women prepare for the hurtful comments. Role playing some of the possible responses the women can make is one way counselors can help women who are infertile be less affected by the comments. Such strategies also provide opportunities for the women to talk about the reasons for their anger and hurt.

Despite counselors' best intentions, infertile women's relationships change, especially with the fertile. For example, pregnant friends of infertile women often try to withhold information about their pregnancies for as long as possible. They may have some guilt because they know how their infertile friend will feel, yet they do not know how to help. Regardless, the fertile and infertile tend to elude each other to avoid the painful feelings that each experiences. Thus, it becomes difficult, if not impossible, to maintain the same level of relationship. Sometimes the change is irreversible.

> We spent Thanksgiving with my family, and my sister just found out she's pregnant. I never thought it would bother me and I'm still amazed it did. . . . I still haven't been able to call her. That's just making me feel even worse, because I'm feeling bad for feeling the way I'm feeling. And I'm feeling guilty about that. It was very difficult. I think the relationship I had with my sister has totally changed. I don't know if it's ever going to be any better. . . . It wasn't entirely me feeling uncomfortable while we were there, I know she was feeling the same way. Then I was feeling bad because she was feeling uncomfortable. I know I was making her feel that way. It was a very tense situation. I felt that I ended up putting a damper on her happiness. And I really didn't want to do that.

Relationships also change with previously infertile women who now become pregnant. As a group, women who are infertile are not genuinely happy for others' pregnancies. Although the previously infertile believe they can provide hope for their infertile friends, the sense of sisterhood that existed has been broken. The pregnant women are not considered members of the club anymore.

Some women also feel estranged from their husbands. Tension between partners escalates when the emotional and marital support necessary to cope with the infertility becomes forced. Many husbands may not seem as deeply motivated toward having a child as do their wives. In such cases, wives may resort to devious behavior in order to have intercourse on the right night. Furthermore, many women feel they must keep up a front. They do not talk about the infertility as much as they would like with their mates because the discussions don't seem to go anywhere. Their spouses become tired of hearing the same things over again without obvious resolution. Some women fear that if they get too upset their husbands will discontinue treatment, as some threaten to do. As a result, women end up walking on eggshells and keeping their feelings hidden.

> Stewart didn't want to know any of the facts. The less that he knew, the easier it was for him to perform on command. He didn't really want all the facts and information.

Women have different reactions to their husbands' infertility. Some are very angry towards their husbands and will have affairs because of this anger. Others are concerned that if they did finally become pregnant by their presumably infertile husbands, that the child would be defective.

In contrast, when the infertility lies with the husband, many wives are very supportive.[7] More than men, women feel a need to present their infertility as a joint problem rather than pointing out the mate as the primary cause. Women find that male infertility can be more difficult to explain to others and more discrediting to the male. Some women become their husbands' protectors and therefore pass the infertility off as "our problem." In some cases, women will take total responsibility for it.

The Woman's Struggle with Herself

Not only do women have to deal with others, they are also struggling with their own feelings. When women lose the ability to bear children, their self-esteem is damaged. Infertile women use words like deviant, defective, and incompetent to describe how they perceive themselves. One woman felt so embarrassed by her body as a result of her infertility that she stopped going to her athletic club. She did not want other women to see her in the locker room. The loss of self-esteem can be so great that infertile women cannot discuss the depth of their feelings, even to others who share the same problem. As many have stated in different ways, "You have to admit failure to some extent."

> I felt that people were looking at me and saying, "What's wrong with you? Why can't you get pregnant?" They weren't, but I felt that they were. I felt . . . degraded. I just felt that there was definitely something wrong with me. I felt as if I weren't as good as anyone else.

Guilt is an emotion commonly experienced.[8] Women who are infertile look to see if there is something they are doing that is causing the infertility. So often, family and friends reinforce the guilt by giving a variety of unsolicited advice strongly suggesting that the women are causing their own infertility, "You are working too hard"; "Maybe you should lose some weight"; "Maybe you should gain weight." Some women take the advice in the hope that it will help them conceive. Others suffer in silence and believe that the infertility is punishment for past sins. They then play the "if only" game.

> "If only I didn't use the pill,"
> "If only I wasn't so heavy,"
> "If only I didn't have premarital sex,"
> "If only I hadn't waited so long to start trying,"
> "If only I didn't have the abortion."

When the infertility is based on the women's problems, there is additional guilt about not giving her partner a child. Many women have been reared to believe that their major role in life is to get married and produce children for their husbands. It is not unusual for a woman to express the desire for her mate to become involved with someone else who could give him a baby.

During the treatment process, many women become obsessed with their hopes of becoming pregnant. The food they eat, the clothes they buy, and even the amount of exercise they do, become contingent upon whether they are preovulatory or premenstrual. As a result, they become nervous, develop problems concentrating on daily activities, and often lose sleep. Research indicates that infertile women find life less interesting, more empty, and more disappointing.[9] They are less satisfied with the amount of success and fulfillment in their lives. Every part of their lives seems to revolve around trying to conceive.

As a result of their infertility, women are uncertain about what in life is within their control. Some women believe that by submitting to all the tests, their bodies and minds are not their own. In contrast, many women feel more in control over their lives when they are going through the testing and treatment. They believe that they are doing something positive to help themselves. But if the treatments fail, and new tests are offered, it is difficult to maintain an optimistic attitude. Women's feelings fluctuate between hope and despair.

As the infertility persists, time becomes more important. Women worry more about the time wasted on lengthy or questionable treatments. They become more aware of their biological clocks and realize that decisions about alternatives need to be considered.

However, successfully coming to terms with infertility is not easy. Regardless of how many doctors are consulted or new techniques attempted, many women remain infertile. Women who realize they have little hope of conception are better able to resolve their infertility. As a result, they can consider alternatives to pregnancy and get on with their lives. However, some women are not as willing to give up. For this group, the decision to terminate treatment is difficult. They are likely to extend time limits that have been set or to convince the physician that they want to go through in vitro fertilization (IVF) one more time. In addition, they delay the end by taking breaks from treatment. The breaks provide a rest, but for many, they also delay the inevitable.

Many women in this position want their physicians to end

treatment. They want the doctor to clearly state there is no hope of their conceiving. However, most physicians find this difficult, believing there is always hope in most cases. To avoid playing God, physicians want their patients to decide on their own how much more treatment they want to pursue. Indeed, with today's technology, the decision is all the more difficult. There are no clear answers.

This is an area where counselors can assist women. By listening to them and to their dilemmas counselors provide women who are infertile an opportunity to problem solve and to make decisions based on their own needs. Because infertility involves so many complicating feelings, it is not easy to sort out true feelings from other's expectations. Counselors can provide women with a safe opportunity to challenge the expectations. Eventually, they can be helped to recognize their own feelings and thus be better able to make decisions regarding future treatments and directions.

In many ways, infertility is like a marathon where the end is unknown. Pace is important since emotional energy is depleted quickly. As a result, there is little time or energy left for anything else. In fact, women describe their life as being "in limbo," "on hold," "dangling," and in the "gray area." Most women who are infertile look forward to the day when their lives will be back to normal. However, in the middle of their struggles with infertility, they find it difficult to believe that day will ever come.

It's like a job. It isn't fun anymore. It's a job with a mission. It's an awful feeling. I just want to go back to the way we were.

2

A Man's Perspective

MY HEART WASN'T IN IT AT FIRST. I went along with Beth because we had agreed early in our relationship that we would have children after five years of marriage. At the time of our initial attempts, I was in graduate school, concentrating on my studies. Yet we proceeded, albeit unsuccessfully. Our families knew, and were probably more excited about the prospect of having a newborn in the family than I was. During the summer vacation after we started trying, my sister and brother-in-law won a big stuffed animal at a carnival for the baby. This only added to the excitement and anticipation. Nobody thought it would be long before both families would have a new infant to indulge.

After a year, the tests began, and I still wasn't into it. In fact, I was embarrassed when I was told the first test would be the postcoital. I went along with whatever Beth wanted. I remember feeling pressured, but there was some excitement also.

After a hysterosalpingogram, Beth became pregnant, right after Thanksgiving. We told people right away and that Christmas was full of excitement. We received several presents for our child-to-be. By this time I was excited about the prospect of being a father, although somewhat nervous.

Several weeks later, Beth had her first miscarriage. I felt so empty and so helpless. Beth was recovering from the anesthesia from the D & C so I had time to kill. I was in a daze for the next several hours. I couldn't wait to see Beth and, when she awoke, I couldn't wait to get her home. We recovered. We shared the loss together, and I think we felt very close; closer than we had in a long time.

We achieved a second pregnancy within a very short time. However, within three months, the physician discovered a blighted ovum, requiring a second D & C. I received a call at work. The doctor told me Beth was hysterical. I felt somewhat embarrassed. Yet, as I think about it now, I get angry at the insensitivity of the doctor. Of course, she was upset—she had just lost her second baby in six months. The empty feeling returned—only worse this time. I was dealing with strong feelings for the first time in my life. I didn't know how to act.

We recovered, again feeling closer than before. We went on summer vacation with my family, including a pregnant sister. The beginning of the week was bad, real bad. Beth was depressed, moody, and easily angered. I was trying to make peace with her, keeping the vacation on a positive note. It culminated with one very bad day. Beth was first angry at my sister, then angry at me. I couldn't understand why. It turned out to be the due date of our first pregnancy. We hugged, Beth cried; I wanted to cry.

We achieved a third pregnancy again. This time we didn't tell anyone, but people knew. There was an unmistakable glow in our faces. However, Beth had a third miscarriage, almost a year to the day of the first. We were somewhat lucky, we were able to stay home as it happened in the middle of the night. I did not want to go to that damn hospital again. The emptiness returned. However, anger also came quickly. I was angry at God for allowing this to happen. I was angry at all the unfairness. By this time, I wanted a child more than anything else in the world.

The testing started quickly, right after the third miscarriage. Because we experienced three miscarriages, genetic testing was done. Never in a million years did I think I would have to put my genes through an evaluation. They passed. Then the specialist and more tests. I put all my energy into being supportive, but sometimes I got fed up. Usually I would take it out on Beth, usually around day 14. It took a while to figure out the pattern.

Years went by and the fighting got worse, then better. At some point we got through all the bad. I think it was when we decided we wouldn't let this thing run our lives. Beth seemed to handle it better as time went on. But I got worse. I got sick and tired of all the pregnant people in the world. I couldn't hold a baby, except for my nieces and nephews. I got angry and depressed every time I saw a pregnant woman and there were many pregnant women around. Again, I was feeling something I never felt before and didn't know quite how to react.

The worse feelings usually came around day 14. We typically

had to have four days of sexual intercourse, spread out over eight days. I would come home from work exhausted, yet it didn't matter, I had to perform. When we were able to successfully fill our quota, we would have several days of calm. However, by day 25 or so, the anticipation would build. We hardly talked about it, yet, we both thought the same thing, "Will this be the month?" Beth would usually tell me she didn't feel optimistic, but I also held out hope. Eventually her period would come and I would be disappointed, angry, and depressed, wondering if we would ever have a child. This cycle went on for many years. Some months were better than others, but they would all end the same, with disappointment, anger, and eventually some despair.

More tests followed and we continued the roller coaster. My role was that of support person. I was comfortable in it, as I was trained to do this. I had the hardest time receiving support. When people would ask how I was doing, I never knew how to respond. I usually said, all right. My true feelings were too difficult to talk about with another person.

My masculinity was never threatened during the process. All sperm counts came back very high. Yet, thinking back now, I was very relieved to know I didn't have a problem. I would cheer wildly with a certain bravado when I'd learn the results of the testing. I don't know how I would react if doctors found a problem with my sperm.

We have a baby now; we adopted. I realized early in the adoption process that carrying on the family genes wasn't the important thing for me, the baby was. With a child I could pass on something more important than my genes—I could pass on my family legacy. The legacy was not a biological legacy, but a sociological one. That legacy that I hope to pass on to my child consists of our families' values and culture.

B earing children does not have the same significance for men as it does for women. For many men, fatherhood is a secondary role. They are socialized to achieve more in the workplace than in the family. Eventually, men do want to have children. However, for the most part, even in our more modern society, rearing a family never has been considered a high priority for many men.

> Boys grow into men without much thought of fatherhood. We think a great deal about school, sports, jobs, careers, earning money, and eventually even about girls, but little, if anything, about babies and nothing about pregnancy (beyond an occasional wishful thought that we might have some opportunity to worry about contraceptives). Never once do we look at pregnant women and imagine that someday we can be involved with that condition. Never once does watching others fawning over a pregnant woman—kidding her about her weight, touching her stomach to feel a kicking baby—create imagined thoughts of the future in our minds. We are taught that when we grow up, we get a job and go to work—always outside the home.[1]

Men associate fertility and having children with the continuation of life, the species, and the family name. Infertility is also a confrontation with death and mortality. These feelings intensify if a man is the only child or even the only male in the family. Culture teaches that men are responsible for carrying on their lineage. Thus, the stress can be unbearable when men believe they can be blamed for the extinction of the family line.

Regardless of the cause of infertility, men tend to be the forgotten partners. Significantly more attention is given to women and their feelings while men take a secondary role, carrying their emotions in silence. Even the medical literature is more heavily weighted toward the women's perspective. However, men's silence cannot be interpreted as a lack of feelings regarding their plight, but instead the result of society's pressure against displaying and discussing them.

We live in a culture that encourages men to be strong and silent, especially when it comes to expressing their feelings. This became evident as we researched this book. Women, for the most part, were willing to talk openly about their experiences and feelings. Not so the men. Furthermore, when men were willing to be interviewed, their wives did most of the talking, even to the point of discussing their husbands' feelings in front of them. At a meeting for infertile couples where the main topic was male infertility, the majority of attendees were women. The men who did attend remained silent, again allowing their wives to speak for them. Thus, it is easy for others to assume that men are either ashamed about what may be their condition or do not care about having children.

Despite their silence, we know that men's reactions to their own infertility are similar to those of women. Their initial experience is shock and disbelief. Some men are insulted that the doctor would suggest that something could be wrong, thinking that the physician has confused his results with those of someone else. In the end, the denial breaks down as the reality of the results becomes apparent.

As occurs with women, men are devastated when they are told that they do have an infertility problem. Infertility goes to the heart of one's sense of self. Men feel that their masculinity is challenged. As is the case with women, men develop low-self esteem and a poor body image. Feelings of being damaged and defective are common. Sometimes rational reasoning diminishes. For example, upon hearing that he was infertile, one man was "afraid I would lose my beard and develop cancer."

> I slipped into a severe depression. Several factors brought this on, but infertility fears were the major catalyst. I withdrew from my wife out of guilt. I was too embarrassed to consult my male friends. I was outraged and felt cheated that infertility was now added to my diabetes, which I had lived with for fifteen years. Where was the justice? It seemed monstrously unfair that we would be denied a child at a time when we were ready to make the commitment. I avoided couples with children, even our best friends. I lost excitement and energy and felt that events were beyond my control. I found myself distracted at work and enduring fits of uncontrollable crying.[2]

Feelings of helplessness are also common to infertile men. For many, this is the first time they have lost the ability to control their lives and choose their destinies.

> I was blinded by the need to achieve this (having a child); it was the only thing in my life up to that point that I could not make happen. I never met an obstacle up to that point that I was not able to conquer. The more energy I put into this, the farther I got behind. I was the victim.

Men generally cope with infertility by blocking it out. They try not to think about it or let themselves feel any emotion related to their problem. However, regardless of how hard they try to block out their feelings, it seems that some aspect of their lives will be negatively affected by the infertility. It could be their marriage, relationships with others, or even their work.

Some men will throw themselves into their work. Unproductiveness in some areas gets compensated for by attempting to overachieve in other areas. For them, work allows them to forget their bad feelings about themselves and also feel good about one aspect of their lives.

In contrast, other men may have difficulty concentrating, become more irritable, and become less productive. Thus, their work becomes problematic, making life more stressful. Infertility becomes just one of a series of problems. As a result, depression becomes common.

The excitement and energy of men's preinfertility days diminish when the diagnosis is confirmed. Many men will withdraw from family and friends, feeling they have lost some status, especially among their fertile peers. Furthermore, they may be too embarrassed to talk about their problem and reveal their true feelings to their male friends. Many choose to suffer in silence, pretending the problem is not a big deal. This loss of status cannot be underestimated. For instance, it is known that some men from the Middle East and Africa may commit suicide when they learn of their own infertility.[3]

> He didn't even realize it, but when he had the sperm count done that was real low, you would see an entirely different person. His attitude was so much different. He walked kind of slumped over, he was really not feeling good about himself. And even though he wouldn't admit it, I could see it. As soon as he had the other count done (which showed great improvement), it was unbelievable. He was standing up straighter. There was just such a difference in his whole attitude, the way he carried himself. He just felt so much better about himself. He didn't even realize how he was. It was amazing to see. He was just like a proud peacock walking around here.

Initially, men cannot understand their wives' emotions when it comes to Mother's Day or learning that their friends are expecting. Gradually the infertility wears them down and they react with the same intensity as their partners.

> My younger brother and his wife were expecting a baby in November of 1983. After the family gathered around to give my dad his Father's Day cards and gifts, my brother's wife and a few of my other relatives presented my brother with "Father-To-Be" cards, thus adding a new item to celebrate on Father's Day. For some reason, I found this extremely difficult to continue to observe. I excused myself and proceeded to walk out to the yard to cry. I was really angry at myself for losing control.[4]

Men are also affected by other couples' pregnancies and children. Like their wives, men will often go out of their way to avoid their friends' and relatives' children. Sometimes pregnant women are hard to avoid.

> I was sitting in a meeting with a person I have been supervising for several years. She had just recently gotten married, so I had never thought of the possibility of her being pregnant. She ended our supervision time by telling me she was three months pregnant, I wanted to reach across the room and strangle her. I thought to myself, "This is great, I have to deal with this person for the next six months, can life get any worse." When I finally spoke, I said something stupid like, "Congratulations—I'm jealous." After she left my office, I sat silently for many minutes, wondering how I would manage this relationship. There had been many (too many) pregnant women at work, but for the most part I was able to avoid them. I knew I would not be able to avoid this one. I was angry and very sad.

The marriage becomes an easy target for the new negative feelings. As with women, guilt is common, resulting in men withdrawing from their partners. They are also angry with themselves at the unhappiness that they feel they are causing their wives.

For men, sex becomes confused with reproduction. A period of impotency is common, with studies showing that about 50 percent of men become impotent within a week of receiving their infertility diagnosis.[5] This generally lasts for a period from one to three months, although in some cases it may go on longer.

Many men, regardless of which partner has the diagnosed problem, experience midcycle impotency, usually caused by the pressure to perform on certain days of the month.

Impotency can be devastating to men. Their worst fears regarding infertility become realized. Feelings about self and about their masculinity hit a new low. Some men will have affairs in order to prove that they continue to be masculine. Sex in the illicit relationship becomes exciting again, as it was in the days before the couple's infertility. In the end, the struggle remains, yet the problems become worse and more complicated.

Counselors, clergy, and other helpers can provide necessary assistance to men who are infertile. Like women, infertile men need to be listened to and to have their feelings validated by others. However, men are most likely to need additional assistance with identifying and expressing their feelings. In general, men are often silent when in comes to their feelings. Men who are infertile are not different and often need help in recognizing their own anger and pain.

If the man is the cause of the infertility, additional help may be needed. These men may have assorted conflicts related to their own identity, their perceived responsibilities regarding maintaining their family's genetic heritage, about their masculinity, or about their life goals in general. Counselors can help these men prevent the conflicts from creating further problems.

Marriages are severely stressed by infertility. Often, men are the forgotten partners as women become the focus of attention. Many men attempt to assist their spouses while denying their own feelings. Their roles as support persons can be overlooked and taken for granted. If their spouses become consumed by their own infertility, men may believe they are becoming less important to their wives. The temptation to look to someone else can be great. Counselors can help these men understand the reasons for their temptations and assist them in deciding how they will effectively handle the associated feelings.

> Her whole life and excitement revolve around whether she is going to have a baby or not. I've really felt left out because of that and I'm not really anticipating it getting better. I feel if she has a kid there's little more need for me except for paying the bills. I don't know, maybe the kid will enhance our relationship together.

But our relationship together is more like friends right now, than it is husband and wife.

It is very possible for me to have an affair. I've had a couple of opportunities. I don't want to have an affair, though; I want somebody to love me. I don't want to have a one-night stand, I want somebody to care for me. . . . She's (wife) withdrawn, she's avoiding me. She doesn't want to go out, she doesn't enjoy things. . . . I want somebody who is enthusiastic about life, someone whom I can support, making me feel that my support is appreciated.

Men are slowly progressing in their responses to infertility. Years ago, most men were minimally involved, even in their own treatment. Today, more men are being treated, albeit reluctantly and with limited success. In addition, more men are becoming actively involved in their wives' treatment. Some are more open about discussing their infertility with others. However, for the most part, men have yet to reach the level of women in their ability to handle infertility and the emotions that are part of the situation.

3

To Want a Child

Be fertile and multiply; fill the earth and subdue it.
Genesis 1:28

T he decision to bear children for many people is voluntary. For the infertile couple, it is a deliberate choice accompanied by emotional strain, physical discomfort, and financial hardship.

> We went to considerable difficulty to have a child. Beth underwent two surgical operations in addition to many less-complicated medical procedures. As a result, she was in severe pain some of the time and in physical discomfort many other times.
>
> We made a serious financial commitment to children as well. Thousands of dollars not covered by insurance were spent on medical procedures. In addition, we committed another ten thousand dollars for adoption. Emotionally, we were on an eight-year roller coaster. There were many highs and lows that included marital disputes, bouts of severe depression, and eight years of anxiety.

With all the struggle and pain we endured to achieve parenthood, it becomes necessary to question our motives. Thankfully, we were not alone. Millions of other couples undergo similar struggles in their quests for children. Couples spend much more than we did on medical procedures. For example, in vitro fertilization can cost up to five thousand dollars per cycle, with couples participating for three or four cycles and still with very little chance of success. In addition, it is known that couples spend up to fifty thousand dollars in the black market to adopt an infant.

It is common for couples to spent fifteen to twenty thousand dollars through legal channels.

The succeeding chapters will explore these hardships in detail so that the reader can begin to appreciate the emotional impact of infertility on the couple. However, in order to understand the depth and breadth of this impact, it first becomes important to understand the significance of wanting children in today's society. The motivation underlying the desire to bear children is complicated and based on historical and social tradition, biological drives, and psychological need.

Fertility in a Historical Context

In ancient cultures, fertility and the ability to bear children played an important role. Couples prayed to the gods of fertility and worshipped statues and paintings of sex organs in order to bring about favor from these gods. They also practiced unusual rites to ward off the evil spirits of barrenness. To determine if a woman might be fertile, they developed strange rituals. One such method used by Hippocrates involved making a mixture of watermelon and human milk, which women would drink. Vomiting showed fertility. If a woman simply belched, she was infertile.[1]

The myth of the stork, still popular today, had its beginning thousands of years ago. The Teutons, an ancient Celtic people, believed that the souls of their unborn children lay in the ponds and feeding grounds of these birds. The stork returning to the same nesting place every year was viewed as an omen of good fortune and fertility. Husbands would build stork shelters on the roof in order to attract the birds so that the spirit children would then be delivered to their home. If a couple did not wish a baby, the man would scare the bird away. To expand one's family one could bait the bird by sprinkling sugar on the windowsill. Some believed the storks actually fathered the children, impregnating women by flying over their houses.[2]

Economic Motivations

In the ancient rituals, there was a strong link between fertility and prosperity. Cave dwelling hunters drew scenes related to fertility consisting of magic rituals practiced to ensure a large herd.[3] In more current times, the rituals included live sexual acts. For instance, European peasants of the nineteenth century would engage in sexual intercourse in the fields to promote an abundant crop.[4]

To the rural families of the past, fertility had a real economic value. The more children a family had, the more laborers available to the parents to work the farm. Even today, it is common for rural families to want more children than do their urban counterparts.[5]

Fertility has another value to rural families. Their heritage, the family farm, has a very special value and is typically passed down through the generations. Recently, many farms are being sold in record numbers at auctions to pay off debts. With the sale, families are losing their heritage. Thus, the farmer is not only letting himself down, and his children who were due to inherit the farm, but also the generations before him who worked the land and had handed it down to him.

Bearing children also provides another asset for families. In some societies, children have a responsibility to care for their elders as they age. Children's responsibility for their parents is a well-known aspect of Asian cultures. Less known is the Hindu tradition, which requires sons to perform certain rituals at their fathers' deaths. Without the rituals, the father would not be able to assume a new form in a subsequent life. Thus children, especially male children, become necessary for the soul's reincarnation.[6]

The Social Context

America is no longer a rural nation. Today, children are no longer an economic asset and are, instead, considered a financial liability. Despite this, we continue to live in a pronatalistic society. Even with the changing roles of men and women, and with more women participating in the job market, having children remains a priority. Current research suggests that 90 to 95 percent of couples want to bear and rear children.[7] Despite the result of urbanization and of women entering the work force, couples continue to want children. However, they are delaying childbirth until they establish their careers. In addition, they are having fewer children. However, the cultural norm that couples should either reproduce or at least want to reproduce continues to dominate our society. Despite our changing values, child-lessness continues to be seen as a form of deviant behavior and a violation of prevailing norms.[8]

There is considerable debate about whether the desire to have children is a learned response or an instinctual need. Bardwick believes that the capacity to bear children is genetically deter-mined and regulated through the hormones.[9] Rossi wants us to believe that a main role of the family system is human continuity through reproduction and child-rearing.[10] On this there can be no debate: children do serve to perpetuate the species.

> One reason I had children was I wanted to take my place in the history of mankind. It was one of the basic universal life experiences. I wanted to feel a part of the continuity of life. I like to think that people have had children for generations before me and will for generations after me.[11]

Children serve to ensure individual immortality as well. It is a common practice from Africa to Iceland to name newborn children after deceased relatives.[12] In more modern times, this practice serves to keep the memory of our ancestors alive. In earlier years, there was the belief that the deceased family member returned in the form of the child. For instance, in French medieval art, "The soul was depicted as a little child who was naked. . . .The dying man breathes the child out through his mouth in a symbolic representation of the soul's departure."[13]

Children also serve to preserve family culture. Values and ethnic traditions are kept alive through our children. Further, parents wish that their children will share values similar to those of the adults.

> I never examined my motivations for wanting children until recently. I always assumed I would be a father. I came from a large family, one brother and three sisters, and remember the good times associated with being part of a family. More impor-tant, I remember the fun my parents seemed to have with their children. Sure, I knew there were difficult times, but for the most part, I watched my parents having fun being parents. When my youngest sister was born, I remember enjoying her infancy and childhood so much. Especially fun was watching her grow up and

learn to respond to the world. I knew I wanted that experience again, with my own children.

It wasn't until I was confronted with the possibility that I might not have my own biological child did I come to understand another motivation for wanting a child. As I got older, the thought that there might not be another person as an heir when I died bothered me. It was important that I left someone behind who could carry on the values that I received from my parents and that they received from my grandparents. As I considered the alternative of adoption, I fully realized it wasn't important to me that my child be biologically connected, just as long as it was someone I could nurture and rear as my own, someone who would carry on my family traditions after I had gone.

Psychological Influences

The value of fertility to families and society has been described. However, bearing and rearing children has special psychological significance as well. Children serve to gratify many conscious and unconscious needs of their parents.

In the psychoanalytic studies of childbearing, pregnancy fulfills the fantasy of the lonely child. The pregnant woman has a companion who is only hers. The baby in utero is always with her and communicates only with her. Like the imaginary friend of childhood, the soon-to-be-born child is a creature of the mother's own making.

> "His Majesty the Baby," as we once fancied ourselves to be. He is to fulfill those dreams and wishes of his parents which they never carried out, to become a great man and a hero in his father's stead. . . . At the weakest point of all in the narcissistic position, the immortality of the ego, which is so relentlessly assailed by reality, security is achieved by fleeing to the child. Parental love, which is so touching and at bottom so childish, is nothing but parental narcissism born again.[14]

For society, children are a vehicle to ensure continuation of the culture. For couples, newborn children provide an opportunity to recreate themselves. They become able, or at least they believe they are able, to create a person in the image they desire, which according to Freud is the person they wish they were.[15] This concept is labeled the deficit-fulfilling motive for parenthood. Parents, through their children, strive to resolve some of their own conflicted life choices and to overcome their own personal deficits. For example, it was common for immigrants or adults who struggled through the depression when younger to want their children to have a better life than theirs. In this sense, children allow parents to live the childhood they dreamed of living, but never did.

Bearing children is also a way to avoid feelings of loneliness. Hoffman and Manis report findings from a multinational survey that explored the reasons adults have children.[16] In the United States, 33 percent of white females believed children could bring them love and companionship.[17] The theories of Durkhiem and Fromm provide a partial explanation for this finding.[18] Accordingly, one way we avoid loneliness is to enter into certain status groups and to participate in secret rituals. For women, pregnancy and childbirth create a ritual. By becoming mothers, women enter a special group and thus have a bond with many others.

> Ever since I was a little girl I knew that I wanted to have children some day. I enjoyed playing with dolls when I was younger. When I was a teenager I spent considerable amounts of time with the children in the neighborhood and enjoyed baby-sitting. I always felt I had a nurturing instinct and was very anxious to have a baby of my own to love, guide and have fun with. I also liked the idea that this child would love me back, unconditionally.
>
> I was never interested in having a career outside the home. To be a wife and mother was my life goal. I wanted to be there when my child was experiencing things for the first time. I looked forward to singing to my child as we went through the day and to comforting my baby when he or she cried.
>
> For a long time I was driven to have a biological child. I was determined that my body was going to overcome any obstacle to achieve pregnancy. When it became obvious that pregnancy might not happen, my reasons for wanting a child became clearer. I didn't need to be pregnant, I wanted a child to love.

Regardless of the motivations behind wanting to have children, parenthood is an important part of the human experience. Human development is about change, with psychological growth occurring as a result of the many crises we experience throughout our lives. As can be attested to by anyone whose has gone through the experience, parenthood represents one such crisis.

The birth of the first child is an important developmental step for couples. For the individuals, having a child marks permanent entry into adulthood and establishes the parents as mature, acceptable members of society. Rearing a child provides challenges and satisfactions never before encountered. In fact, data suggest that adults of both sexes believe that becoming a parent is the most significant event defining adult status.[19]

Most parents are at a stage where motivation for creativity and productivity are at their highest levels. Children provide a means of expressing this need. For women, pregnancy has been observed as a period of maturation and integration. Motherhood represents a progressive development culminating in the mother–child relationship.

> Giving birth was like no other experience I have had. Giving to an infant pushed me beyond whatever I imagined my capacity for giving was, and seeing my children grow and develop is uniquely satisfying.[20]

For couples, birth marks becoming a family. Couples move from being a pair to a threesome and thus, for the first time, a real system.

The Biology

We also have explored some of the motivations behind the need to have children. It is complicated and based on complex combinations of economic necessity, biological imperatives, and psychological need fulfillment. Indeed, understanding infertility requires knowledge of the interaction between psychology and biology. We also have explored some of the motivations associated with wanting children. Let us not forget the biology of producing children, because it is an integral part of understanding infertility and the emotions experienced by the infertile couple.

The Fertilization Process

Remember the story of the stork? Today, this story can often satisfy a child curious about the origins of babies, but it cannot appease us. How simple it might have been to drink a potion to determine fertility and accept the results. Or to build a nest for a bird and hope he makes it his home. The ancient cultures did not understand human reproduction as we do today. However, even with our knowledge derived from modern technology, conception is far more complex than we can imagine.

Let us first take a look at the female reproductive system in very simplified terms. Girls are born with ovaries containing 300,000 to 400,000 follicles or immature eggs. At puberty, around twelve years of age, girls begin menstruation.

The typical menstrual cycle is 28 days. The first day of menstruation is called day 1; and day 14 is the approximate time of ovulation. Menstrual cycles can vary, so pinpointing ovulation is sometimes difficult.

During the first half of the cycle, a follicle, or sometimes more than one, begins to mature under the influence of estrogen. At the same time, the follicle moves toward the surface of the ovary. The uterine lining, called endometrium, is thickening in preparation to receive a fertilized egg. The cervical mucous, also under the influence of estrogen, turns clear and elastic, in order to be receptive to potential sperm.

When the follicle does rupture, around day 14, the egg is trapped in the oviduct at the end of the Fallopian tube and begins its five- to seven-day journey down the tube. Normally, conception takes place in the top third of the Fallopian tube, nearest the ovary. The ruptured follicle, now called the corpus luteum, releases progesterone causing the endometrium to secrete nourishment for the fertilized egg. If conception has occurred, implantation takes place in the uterus. If all is successful, the fertilized egg becomes an embryo, then a fetus, and finally a newborn infant.

If the follicle is not fertilized, the corpus luteum continues to produce hormones for twelve more days. As these hormone levels drop, the lining is no longer nourished, bringing the onset of menstruation. After menstruation, which can last for three to seven days, a new cycle begins.

The male reproductive system may seem less complicated, but in fact many problems can occur. To begin, the male's external sex organs consist of the penis and two testes, or testicles, which are connected by a system of tubes.

The testes contain the hormone testosterone and also the seminiferous tubules that produce sperm cells. After initial development, the sperm cells empty into a coiled, tubular structure called the epididymis for further maturation. The epididymis joins the vas deferens, a straight, tubular structure. From the vas deferens, which is in the abdomen, the cells travel through the penis via the urethra. Before the sperm enters the urethra, it is stored near the seminal vesicle. Semen, which consists of the sperm, fluids from the prostate, and other secretions, leaves the body during an ejaculation. The movement is caused by a series of muscular contractions of the tube known as peristalsis. The first part of the ejaculation carries the most sperm, as many as 500 million. But only tens of thousands gain access to the uterus, and only one will penetrate the egg and fertilize it.

For conception to occur, the sperm have to meet the egg at ovulation. The sperm have a life of seventy-two hours; the egg is viable from twenty-four to forty-eight hours. Women are most likely to conceive if intercourse takes place the day before, the day of, and the day after ovulation. For conception to take place, sexual intercourse should occur during this time so that the sperm can swim up the cervix through good, elastic cervical mucous. With everything working optimally, there is a 25 percent chance of conception in any one month. This percentage decreases with age. Furthermore, in one year 80 percent of couples who attempt pregnancy will conceive.[21]

Deciding to Have Children

In years past, the timing of the first child was straightforward and required little decision making on the part of the married couple. Birth control methods were rudimentary with high rates of failure. In addition, there were strong religious and social mores that prevented the existing methods from being effectively utilized. Many couples would, by necessity, have children shortly after marriage.

For couples today, the decision to begin a family is more complex. With the development of more effective, readily available birth-control methods, couples have more control over their reproductive lives. With the changed status of women in society, and with the prevalence of dual career marriages, parenting roles have become less defined. Thus, couples have many factors to consider. We will explore some of the issues in the decision-making process.

First, the individuals involved have to determine if they are psychologically ready for children. The birth of the first child results in a significant increase of responsibility to the parents. With a newborn comes change and disruption. There are more financial responsibilities and some loss of personal freedom. Individuals need to decide if they are ready to have another human being be totally dependent on them.

Second, couples have to decide if they feel the marriage is ready for the stress of children. Couples spend the initial stages of marriage adjusting to each other, getting used to different habits and customs, and learning the others' likes and dislikes. With children, couples have less time for each other and spend more time involved in children-oriented activities. If one partner is not prepared for the change, the results can be disruptive to the newly created family.

Career is another issue that needs to be considered. In the past, roles were more clearly defined—men worked and women stayed home to parent. For many modern couples, both members are committed to their careers. Thus, with a new child jobs will be disrupted. For women, childbirth means that there will be lost time from work. For men, especially those who plan to share parenting responsibilities, there will, by necessity, be more disruptions to work and career. There may never be a good time in a career to have children, but there are probably times that are better than others.

Finally, biology is a consideration. Although women do bear children into their forties, the biological clock is real. Two issues are pertinent here. First, fertility does decrease as one gets older.[22] Thus, the longer women wait to bear children, the greater the likelihood that there will be difficulty with conception. Endometriosis has been called the "career woman's disease" because it is more prevalent in women who delay childbirth.

Additionally, the chances of birth defects increase with age.[23] For example, the risk of having a child afflicted with Down's Syndrome increases for women over thirty-five. All couples may not be prepared for the challenge of a special child.

Although couples may not consider all these options when they decide to have children, the decision, for many, is rational and planned. When the decision is made to conceive, couples assume that the process is under their control. Indeed, until this time, many have made a considerable effort to prevent pregnancy. Most, having been successful in their-birth control methods, now expect to have an instant family. However, for 15 to 20 percent of couples, the expectations are not fulfilled and, for many, their dreams are crushed.[24] They are diagnosed as being infertile. The remainder of the book will explore how their lives will be affected by this diagnosis.

Considerations for Counseling

Children hold a place of importance in our society. This chapter has explored some of the historical, social, and psychological backgrounds for our need to bear children. For the counselor working with couples, the information can be useful in several ways:

1. When working with couples, counselors, clergy, and other helpers can assume that most couples, but not all, will want to bear children sometime in their marital relationship.
2. If a couple has decided to remain child-free, there will be social stigma attached to this decision. Counseling might be necessary to assist couples who are dealing with the stigma.
3. For couples who decide they want children, there is information available that can be useful to couples when they begin their attempts to conceive. Counselors can also help

couples to set realistic expectations about their probability of success.

4. For counselors who work with infertile couples, this chapter provides a foundation for understanding why children are important. The motivations are rooted in historical and social tradition and strong psychological need. With this foundation, counselors will better understand the depth of emotion that will be described in the subsequent chapters.

4

Beginning the Struggle with Infertility

AS MONTHS WENT BY and I still wasn't pregnant, I wandered into a bookstore looking for something that might tell me that everything was all right. I was very discreet because I didn't want anyone to know what I was looking at. Suddenly, the word jumped off the page at me and my heart stopped: INFERTILITY. Yes, I fit the definition.

I was too embarrassed and angry to buy the book that day. But later on, once I had calmed down, I realized that I might need a little more information than I already had. Maybe we weren't timing things correctly. What was that I had heard about cervical mucous and the basal body temperature? Who would have thought it would be this complicated?

Infertile—the word itself carries a stigma. For men, it's an assault on their masculinity. For women, infertility is equated with barrenness, which history tells us is a curse.

Initially, when couples suspect that there is a problem they feel alone. They think that they are the only ones whose bodies are failing them. However, statistics show this is not the case. Fifteen percent of couples today have an infertility problem.[1] For the 28 million people who are of reproductive age, that equals 4.5 million men and women. The percentage may not sound like a significant number—it translates into one couple in six. However, at the next party you attend with eleven other couples, remember that out of that group, two couples may have a problem with infertility.

Women in their early twenties have a 20 to 25 percent chance of conceiving in any given month. However, this percentage drops with age. In the late twenties, the chances of becoming pregnant are 15 to 20 percent. In the early thirties the odds are 10 to 15 percent, and in the late thirties couples have an 8 percent chance of conception each month.[2] Thus, even for couples not diagnosed as infertile, initial attempts to conceive will most likely be unsuccessful and filled with moments of disappointment and frustration.

Before seeking medical help, couples can do a few simple things on their own to improve their chances of conceiving. Becoming aware of the woman's body and cycle is a good place to start.

According to Regina Matties, a nurse practitioner who has worked with infertile couples for thirteen years:

> Some people are not knowledgeable at all (about basic physiology). Just the basic timing, no lubricant, people don't know that unless they've gone to a natural family-planning class or something like that. . . . Some people try to pick "the day" and not have intercourse the rest of the month. It's basic knowledge. . . . Some still think they are ovulating on day 14 even if they have a thirty-five-day cycle, they don't know they're ovulating on day 21.

The timing of intercourse around ovulation is very important. Thus, pinpointing ovulation is the first step in increasing the probabilities of conception. Ovulation usually occurs around the woman's midcycle. The midcycle is usually fourteen days counting backward from the first day of her period. So in the average twenty-eight-day-cycle, ovulation should occur on day 14. In a thirty-eight-day-cycle, ovulation should happen on day 24, and on day 11 in a twenty-five-day cycle.

Ovulation predictor test kits provide another method of determining ovulation. These kits are used at home and predict ovulation one to two days in advance. When using the ovulation predictor kit, the woman tests her urine for her body's leutinizing hormone (LH) for several consecutive days before the suspected day of ovulation. Just before ovulation, the LH surges, and the color of the test strip in the kit changes, signaling impending ovulation.

The basal body temperature or BBT test is probably the most common test used for determining the approximate time of ovulation. When using the BBT method, women take their temperature each morning and plot it on graph paper. The temperature must be taken before getting out of bed when the body is at total rest, hence the word basal. A regular thermometer may be used, but we recommend a basal thermometer because it is easier to read.

The body's normal temperature is 98.6° F. However, at rest, the temperature can be as low as 97° F. After ovulation, the basal temperature is approximately 98° F. The hormone progesterone raises the body's temperature, causing the slight increase. The BBT chart should show a slight dip followed by a gradual rise. Ovulation will occur anytime between the dip and the peak of that rise.

The basal body temperature chart provides several important types of information. First, the graph shows the occurrence of ovulation by a rise in temperature. When the BBT chart does not show a rise in temperature, there is reason to believe that ovulation did not occur. The BBT chart also highlights the length of the luteal phase in the menstrual cycle. If menstruation occurs earlier than twelve days after the rise in temperature, a condition called luteal phase defect may be present. Finally, if the temperature remains elevated for several days past the expected date of menstruation, pregnancy may have occurred.

The cervical mucous should be examined along with the BBT chart. In the beginning of the menstrual cycle, the cervix is closed and produces little mucous. As ovulation approaches, the cervix opens and a large amount of watery mucous becomes evident. The consistency of this mucous changes when ovulation becomes imminent. When the mucous becomes clear and elastic, ovulation is most likely one to two days away. It is at this point that the mucous is most receptive to the sperm. Just after ovulation the cervix closes and the quality of the mucous changes. It becomes sticky, thick, and cloudy and traps the sperm, preventing them from entering the cervix.

For pregnancy to occur, sexual intercourse needs to take place around the time of ovulation. As the methods described provide only estimates for ovulation, the charts should be used only as guides. After couples use the charts for several months, certain trends become evident. By interpreting the charts and examining the cervical mucous, couples should be able to estimate the time of ovulation with some degree of accuracy.

To maximize chances for conception, couples should have intercourse starting at least four days before the expected ovulation date. Intercourse should occur every other day, continuing until several days after ovulation. The sperm count needs time to return to a normal range, so having intercourse more often can be detrimental. The sperm are able to survive in the Fallopian tubes for up to seventy-two hours, so more frequent intercourse serves no purpose. If a couple waits to have intercourse until the temperature has risen, they are most likely past their fertile time for that month.

Seeking Medical Assistance

Initially, women usually discuss their fertility concerns with their gynecologists. For the most part, the gynecologist is someone a woman visits on a regular basis, has developed a trustful relationship with, and should feel comfortable talking to about her infertility. Depending on the woman's age, the physician may not be concerned until the couple has unsuccessfully attempted to conceive for a full year. However, because fertility does decrease with age, some physicians may begin testing after six months for women over thirty years of age, and after only three months when over thirty-five years.[3]

Primary infertility is defined as the failure to conceive after one year of regular intercourse without the use of contraception. Secondary infertility is the failure to conceive following one or more births.[4] Thus, couples should consider seeking medical help after one year of unsuccessful attempts to conceive. Fifty to 60 percent of infertile couples can be successfully treated if they have expert medical care.[5] However, many couples will delay because, in their minds, seeking medical help makes the infertility all too real.

> The first time I got my bill and saw the diagnosis "Infertility," it was surprising. Even if you know you have a problem before you

go, seeing it on that piece of paper, or having him tell you that this is what it is, it makes it very tough to avoid from that point on.

There are many things that can go wrong with the female reproductive system that contribute to infertility. Research shows that in women 30 percent of infertility is cause by hormonal problems, 20 percent by endometriosis, 30 percent by structural problems such as blocked tubes, and 10 percent by immunological problems between the male and female. The final 10 percent is unexplained.[6] Since the focus of this book is psychological, not biological, we will not detail all the ways fertility is impeded. There are many good references given that do this. However, a brief discussion is in order.

Unless the cause of the infertility is known, the evaluation process begins with women charting their basal body temperature. In addition, couples note on the chart each time they have sexual intercourse. Thus, for the first time, couples realize that their infertility results in an invasion of their personal lives. However, most are willing to do whatever it takes to have a baby.

In the beginning, couples believe they are doing something positive to resolve their problem. Moreover, as soon as they can find the exact time of ovulation on the graph, and program intercourse accordingly, they feel pregnancy will come easily. Many soon realize the cure for infertility is not that simple.

At first, charting is done compulsively, but with the idea that it can be abandoned after a few months. Not a day is missed. As time passes, the charting becomes habitual and the graph becomes committed to memory. They do not refer to the days of the month in the normal manner, but instead to day 7 or day 14. The graphs have now become the "Bible according to ovulation." Many couples continue to chart for years with the same conviction.

Because couples' sexual lives are monitored so closely, sexual excitement becomes diminished as time passes. Furthermore, as ovulation approaches, the pressure to have sex on schedule increases, particularly for men. Sexual problems occur. Some women may have little sympathy for their partners when they are unable to perform on cue. Indeed, if a woman is undergoing the bulk of the treatment, she may expect her mate to happily fulfill his part of the bargain. Thus, marital conflicts become common.

When charting for ovulation does not bring conception, additional tests are necessary. One of the initial tests conducted will be the postcoital test or Simms-Huhner, test. This is used to evaluate the sperms' interaction with the cervical mucous. The test must take place around the woman's midcycle, when the cervical mucous is most receptive to the sperm.

For this simple procedure, the couple engages in intercourse. After several hours, the woman goes to the physician's office to have the quality of the mucous checked. The procedure is painless as the doctor aspirates a small amount of cervical mucous, to determine if it is clear and elastic. The mucous is then examined under a microscope to observe if the sperm are able to survive in the environment. Some women produce hostile mucous, which kills the sperm. At the same time, the number of sperm are counted and the motility evaluated. This test does not replace a separate semen analysis. Because the doctor may want to follow up on questionable results, or if the couple's timing was not quite right, the postcoital test may be repeated over several cycles.

Although the test is physically painless, emotionally it can be draining. Couples need to have sexual relations at unusual times, usually in the morning. This often causes many to lose sleep, which only adds to the problem of performance anxiety. The postcoital test can also be embarrassing because couples are not used to others' knowing about their sexual activities. Many think that the staff are grading their performance.

One couple was told to have intercourse from six to eight hours before their morning appointment for a postcoital test. The woman was also told not to shower before her appointment.

> I must have had the test scheduled a hundred times. . . . It was always either I wouldn't ovulate, or part of the problem was they were always scheduling it for first thing in the morning. So I was setting the alarm clock for two or three o'clock in the morning and then saying, " Ok, honey, come on." He would not be very receptive to the idea. So for all of those different reasons, it never occurred. . . . Part of me is wondering, "Did I never have the test because it really bothered me?" . . . I've always been one where

when you do have your exam you shower the second before you go . . . and you still feel uncomfortable. And then having to have sex, be told you can't shower afterwards—it really bothered me. Maybe because I didn't want it to happen, that's why it didn't happen.

Blood tests for men and women are also part of the initial workup. These tests show the presence of certain infections, evaluate hormone levels, and assess the functioning of important organs and glands. Although blood tests can be time-consuming and expensive, it is important that they be conducted. In the infertility workup, drawing blood is one of the least invasive procedures, and it can also be the most informative.

Another test that is often required for women is the endometrial biopsy. On one of the last days of the menstrual cycle, a tiny piece of lining is removed from the uterus. The procedure can be done in the gynecologist's office. The biopsy can be somewhat uncomfortable, so to ease the pain, some physicians use a mini paracervical block.

The endometrial biopsy evaluates several components of women's menstrual cycle. The test evaluates the level of progesterone in the endometrium. Progesterone needs to be secreted in a quantity sufficient to build a good endometrial lining, which is necessary to sustain pregnancy. If the results confirm that ovulation has occurred, the date of ovulation in the menstrual cycle is also revealed. The results are compared to the BBT chart to determine if the date of ovulation according to the graph corresponds to the date provided by the biopsy.

Ovulatory Problems

Anovulation or irregular ovulation can be caused by several things. Polycystic ovarian disease or Stein-Leventhal syndrome causes hormonal imbalances that affect ovulation. These imbalances cause multiple cysts to form in the ovaries. Birth-control pills may also hinder the resumption of ovulation.

Many women take ovulation for granted. They assume that their bodies are ovulating because "it is such a simple task."

When they discover that they are not ovulating they "feel sad that their body had such a difficult time." Most dread the thought of using drugs because it is "unnatural." But when medication is prescribed, many have high expectations of what it will do.

> Expecting I was going to have trouble really mediated my expectations. But it still went through my mind, "How long is it going to be?" You get tired of taking your temperature for a year without even seeing a chance, your temperature never even going up. . . . The first time he put me on it (Clomid) he didn't put me on a high enough dose, so I didn't ovulate. So he went to 100 mg. and the second month on 100 mg. I got pregnant. . . . When I didn't get pregnant the first time (on the right dose) I was disappointed, more disappointed than I had been the whole previous year. Because I thought they had put me on this (Clomid), it corrects the problem, it's going to work. I was much more expectant that first month of being on Clomid than I had been the whole prior year, which was really funny. I have that feeling now, especially having gotten pregnant, that I feel if I go on Clomid in two or three months I better be pregnant. I'll be really blown away if that doesn't happen.

If anovulation or irregular ovulation is the problem, clomiphene is the first choice of treatment. Clomiphene citrate, or Clomid, is the most common and safest of the fertility drugs. Clomid is not a hormone, but tricks the body into making more of its own hormones. The drug works on the hypothalamus to block estrogen and increase follicle-stimulating hormone (FSH) production. Clomid is administered in tablet form, usually with a shot of human chorionic gonadotropin (HCG) to ensure the rupture of the follicles. Clomid can be a very effective treatment. With treatment, 80 percent of the anovulatory patients begin to ovulate. About 40 to 50 percent will become pregnant.[7] However, there are also side effects.

Many patients complain of depression, headaches, nausea, vomiting, hot flashes, insomnia, and severe mood swings. Probably the most annoying side effect is the emotional reaction. One woman thought she "was going crazy" and sought psychiatric help as a result. Her physician had told her that Clomid had no side effects. Naturally she was very upset when she was told that Clomid was indeed the drug causing her irritability. Some women feel obliged to tell their friends and co-workers that they are taking medication because of their moodiness and irritability. The severe mood swings caused by the drug only add to the emotionality of infertility.

Hysterosalpingogram

Another procedure used in the infertility workup is the hysterosalpingogram. This procedure, which provides a picture of the uterus and tubes, determines if the Fallopian tubes are open and if there may be damage or abnormalities in the uterus. The procedure, which involves injecting a radiopaque dye through the cervix into the uterus, is completed by either the gynecologist or a radiologist. X rays are then taken. If the dye spills out into the abdominal cavity, the tubes are considered normal. The procedure can be somewhat painful, with a few cramps lingering afterward.

> I had a one hysterosalpingogram. That was enough for me. I don't think you could even talk me into doing it again. They told me, "This might be a little uncomfortable." I almost jumped off the table.

With the hysterosalpingogram, the results are known immediately. Furthermore, small obstructions may be dislodged when the test is done. Occasionally, pregnancy will occur shortly after the completion of the procedure, as it did with us.

Male Infertility

While these initial tests are being done on the woman, the man should also begin a workup. Statistics show that 35 percent of the infertility problems lie solely with the female, and 35 percent with the male. A problem may be found with both in 20 percent of cases. Only about 10 percent of infertility is unexplained.[8]

There are many causes of infertility in men. These include blockage of sperm ducts, hormonal problems related to the endocrine system, infections, especially involving sexually transmitted diseases, and genetic factors such as Klinefeltcrs syndrome. However, each of these problems accounts for only a relatively small percentage of cases. In more than half of the male infertility cases, the problem cannot be identified.[9] This is termed "ideopathic oligospermia."

Because of the biology of the male reproductive system, i.e, the accessibility of the penis and testicles, the evaluation of infertility in males is less complicated than for females. Nevertheless, the evaluation and treatment procedures men endure can still be frustrating, difficult, and at times embarrassing.

As previously stated, men may have some blood work completed to check for the presence of hormonal abnormalities and infections. In addition, the postcoital test will give some indication of the quality of his sperm. However, this is not a substitute for a detailed semen analysis.

Semen analysis

The semen analysis should be conducted by a qualified urologist or andrologist. The procedure is painless but somewhat embarrassing. A sperm sample is produced by masturbation. Many men feel that the test is a humiliation. Initially, they may resist having the test done and end up making the appointment with considerable trepidation. Most men are fortunate enough to be able to bring the sample from home. However, when fresh specimens are needed, a sample produced at the office or lab may be required, making the procedure that much more stressful.

Some men, either because of the embarrassment and stress involved, or because of religious convictions, cannot masturbate into a jar. In cases such as these, alternative methods are necessary. For example, couples may collect the specimen as part of coitus interruptus. Special condoms are made that also can be used to collect a sample for analysis.

> I don't think I could masturbate into a jar. I don't think I could excite myself enough to produce sperm. I don't care if you show me a magazine of nude girls. . . . I just can't see myself getting myself excited to the point of producing a specimen. If my wife was in the room with me I'd have no trouble producing a spec-

imen (coitus interruptus), but to be in a room by myself, I know I couldn't do it.

Four areas of the semen sample are evaluated. The amount of semen gets measured and the number of sperm counted. A fertile male has around 20 to 100 million sperm per cubic centimeter of fluid. The normal volume is two to five cc's. Furthermore, the motility or activity of the sperm is observed. It is expected that at least 60 percent of the sperm are moving after two hours.[10] If the analysis shows a good count, but poor motility, the specimen would be further examined for clumping (agglutinization), indicating an immunologic reaction. Finally, the shape of the sperm and the appearance of the semen are evaluated. Several analyses may be required for the physician to make a proper diagnosis.

Because so many factors can affect the count temporarily, the test is usually repeated two or three times. Factors such as illness and medication can affect the sperm count for periods up to three months. In addition, some believe that a low count might also be caused by exposure to whirlpools and saunas or possibly from wearing tight underwear. Thus it is important to understand that a diagnosis of low sperm count cannot be made until several specimens have been examined over a period of three months to ensure that the results are consistent and to rule out temporary conditions.

A health history is also a very important part of the male workup. Such illnesses as mumps and diabetes have a specific effect on male fertility. With appropriate treatment, these problems can usually be corrected.

Sometimes fertility drugs, such as clomiphene, human menopausal gonadotropin (HMG), and human chorionic gonadotropin (HCG) are used to improve sperm counts. These drugs are indicated when hormonal abnormalities are discovered, but are also utilized when the cause is unknown. Drug therapy for males is a controversial area as there is little scientific evidence that these drugs are effective for males. There is usually only a 20 percent chance of successful impregnation using drug therapy.[11] Some couples feel it is not worth the annoyance, while others feel drugs are their only hope.

Varicoceles

Structural problems are also associated with male infertility. They are the easiest of the causes to identify, requiring a physical examination of the male sex organs. The varicocele, which is a varicose vein of the testicle, is the most common structural problem. Varicoceles occur in 10 to 15 percent of all men and cause low sperm count in about 25 percent of all infertile men.[12] The relationship between the varicocele and infertility is currently unknown. However, some believe that the increased blood that pools in the scrotum as a result of the varicocele causes the temperature to rise, resulting in a reduction of sperm production.

Varicoceles can be treated radiologically or surgically. Surgery can be performed on an outpatient basis, with either general or local anesthesia. Surgery involves making an incision in the abdomen and tying the internal spermatic vein. Sperm counts improve in about 75 percent of the cases.[13]

Although the procedure is relatively easy and straightforward, many men become panic-stricken at the thought of surgery. Many will want a second opinion because they are "petrified of going under the knife." As is the case with any surgery, a second opinion is recommended.

The Emotions of Infertility

For us, childbirth, like other aspects of our lives, was to be a well-planned event. All relevant aspects were taken into account, career development and achievement, financial security, amount of time needed to become familiar with each other, and age. Considerable attention was given in the earlier stages of our marriage to control fertility in order to assure that a pregnancy did not occur before the timing was right. We still remember, with some humor, that one time Beth missed her period and how anxious that made us. Five years into our marriage, we decided we were ready, and proceeded with the task of trying to produce a child. Pregnancy was like every other event in our lives together, a goal to be achieved. Like other goals, we felt, with some confidence, we could achieve it with little difficulty. Developmentally, we believed we were ready for the next stage of adult life.

After several months of unsuccessful attempts, the excitement changed to surprise at the difficulty, which turned to frustration and disappointment at the failed attempts. What was to be an exciting process of attempting conception turned into a chore. As the stress became greater, fights became more prevalent and sex was no longer fun and exciting. When relatives or acquaintances asked us if we had any children, the answer "No" more often than not got stuck in our throats. At some point, and it is difficult to know just when, we realized we were infertile.

As time progressed, we felt more and more alone. Greater amounts of conversation at gatherings centered on pregnancies, childbirth, and finally rearing children. We wanted so badly to join in these conversations as one of the experts on parenting, but fate would not permit it. There seemed to be more and more baby showers. Sometimes we were lucky to have reasons not to attend, other times we were not. What was to be an important developmental milestone became a personal crisis for both of us.

Infertility is a major life crisis. In today's society, where couples plan all their life events, greater numbers find that this is one aspect of their lives that they cannot control. What seems to happen so easily for others, sometimes by accident, will now become the center of infertile couples' lives. For many, infertility is the most stressful crisis they will experience.

The emotions associated with infertility are as much a part of the condition as are the physical components. Research shows that 25 to 40 percent of patients who attend infertility clinics report emotional symptoms of clinical significance.[14] Past beliefs held that emotional conditions contributed to infertility in many cases. However, those studies relating emotional functioning with infertility did not take into account the degree to which infertility caused the emotional turmoil. Current findings are inconclusive about the contribution emotions play in continued infertility. One thing is clear, the emotional responses are inevitable, and the struggle infertile couples have with their emotions is as hard as, if not harder than, any other component associated with the condition.

Couples learn early in their infertility that emotional reactions are not confronted just once, but are something they struggle with constantly. Anger, depression, periods of intermittent hope followed by despair, and continuous anxiety are just some of the emotions experienced. The longer infertility remains a problem, the more prominent a part the emotions will play in their lives. Some couples experience these emotions for the first time in their lives and do not believe they can handle them.

Three models have been proposed to describe the emotional components of infertility. Barbara Eck Menning, a pioneer in counseling the infertile, uses a stage model.[15] According to Menning, couples experience a common pattern of seven emotions in a predictable order. Based on her extensive work, she believes couples first act surprised when they initially confront their difficulty in conceiving. Surprise is followed by denial, anger, isolation, guilt, and grief as the infertility continues to be problematic. Finally, at some point, couples come to a resolution about their infertility. Looking back at the scenario given above, some of the emotions described by Menning are apparent.

Hill views infertility as a series of traumas confronted each month.[16] Throughout the struggle, stress is felt to varying degrees. All infertile couples experience emotional side effects as a result of their infertility. What varies is the degree of the severity of the side effects. Hill makes a case for classifying infertility as post-traumatic stress disorder based on the following:

1. The inability to have children is outside the range of the human experience of most of the general population and is sustained by the couple as private and isolating, thus causing great distress.
2. The trauma is experienced over and over again each month with the onset of the menstrual cycle, a verification that the goal of having a child has failed. This continues month after month and can go on year after year.
3. Couples attempt to avoid stimuli that remind them of their loss, such as movies, children's clothing and maternity departments at shopping malls, baby showers, christenings, diaper displays and baby food aisles in supermarkets, television commercials that use children to sell products, and even sexual intimacy with their partners.
4. The most stable people who experience infertility report these common problems: a loss of interest in activities and hobbies which they formerly engaged in; a loss of sleep;

irritability, rage, inability to concentrate, and a general loss of enthusiasm about life.

Fleming views infertility as a chronic medical condition.[17] In this approach, couples never fully resolve the infertility. Even after pregnancy, the infertility becomes part of couples' history and cannot be forgotten. This history becomes revived when attempts are made to conceive an additional child. Thus, the goal for infertile couples is to learn to cope and adapt to their condition.

From our point of view, all the models have something to offer. Certainly, couples regularly confront the emotions described so adequately by Menning. Whether they occur in the sequence suggested is a question best left to researchers. However, the degree to which couples resolve their infertility is less clear. As Fleming notes, couples constantly struggle with their condition. Some people do learn to cope and adapt to their condition. They may not allow the infertility to affect other aspects of their lives. To that degree the infertility gets resolved. However, the feelings continue to exist and couples continue to confront them from time to time in various degrees.

In the initial stages of infertility, understanding the emotional components is critical to the mental health of the couple. They soon realize that dealing with the emotional aspects of their diagnosis is not to try to make the feelings go away—they don't. Successful adjustment means minimizing the negative effects, handling them when they become prominent, and having some control over them so they do not become totally disruptive to other areas of the couple's lives.

Many times, people around the infertiles diminish the importance of the feelings experienced. Statements like:

> "Relax!"
> "You are working too hard, go on a vacation and you'll get pregnant," or
> "You don't know how lucky you are, children can be very difficult"

are never helpful and only make people angry. It is important that those who want to provide emotional support to infertile couples assure them that although the struggle with infertility will be difficult, they can and will survive.

Suggestions for Improved Emotional Functioning

Throughout, we have provided some ways in which counselors, clergy, and other helping professionals can assist people who are infertile. There are some additional suggestions that couples might find useful as they adapt to their infertility in these initial stages:

1. Help them acquire information about infertility. The most difficult part of infertility is couples' confusion about their bodies. On one hand, people who are infertile feel well physically, but on the other, there is something wrong with their bodies that is causing the infertility. Emotional responses to infertility are related to the degree to which people have knowledge about the causes and proper treatment of their condition.

   Ambiguity is a major issue for couples.[18] Uncertainty regarding the causes of infertility leads to general anxiety, disequilibrium and poorer psychological adjustment to the infertility. Research shows that people who do not secure information tend to believe their problems are not solvable.[19] As a result, they are apt to feel helpless and out of control and thus give up. Self-esteem suffers. In contrast, specific reading that helps people who are infertile gain knowledge about themselves and their environment is related to facing and solving problems, relieving stress, and developing insight. The knowledge gained by reading will help couples know what to expect during the evaluation and treatment of their condition. In addition, they will be able to develop realistic expectations about success rates of procedures. Reading also enables couples to know when the doctor is following acceptable routines regarding diagnosis and treatment. Despite what people think to the contrary, doctors like knowledgeable patients.

2. Help them take care of their physical needs. Frustration and depression are some of the emotions experienced by

couples. It is important that they not allow themselves to succumb to their depression, give up, and allow the infertility to take over their lives. Instead, couples need to pay extra attention to caring for themselves. For example, eating well and following recommended nutritional guidelines prevent the body from deteriorating.

Individuals who are infertile also need to stay active. When we are able to engage in satisfying projects, the work helps keep our minds off our problems. Furthermore, the sense of accomplishment that comes with the completion of concrete tasks increases self esteem.

Finally, a regular exercise routine will help fight the loss of esteem and feelings of depression that surface. Exercise increases feelings of relaxation, something very important to those who struggle with anxiety throughout their infertility.

3. Help them accept the emotional components as part of their infertility. People who are infertile may experience intense emotions for the first time in their lives. Emotions are part of the infertility. As such, couples should be prepared for the rage, depression, anxiety, that will surface. It is critical that they are not frightened of these emotions. People need permission to feel what they feel and express what they need to express. By accepting these emotions as part of the infertility package, couples can get on with the business of adapting to their infertility.

5

Advanced Infertility

Changing to a Specialist

For some infertile couples, treatment by the gynecologist may be all that is needed to achieve pregnancy. If initial tests indicate that the problem is routine, the physician may feel confident enough to treat the problem. However, many couples require more complex treatment and need to know when to move on to a specialist.

It is common for women to have special relationships with their gynecologists. For many women, the physician has been a confidant and someone they trust with their most personal problems. Their gynecologist is the person they hoped would deliver their babies. Patients tend to be very loyal. For women to tell their doctors they want to seek the opinion of an expert in infertility can be stressful and awkward.

> He (gynecologist) pretty much dragged his feet. Finally, after all that time (three years) he sent us to an infertility specialist. . . . We were just going along with the routine of doing things that he was suggesting to do. And looking back . . . I should have, back then, just said, "I want to go to a specialist and get all this done as fast as possible." He never really found anything.

Physicians may also have problems referring patients to specialists. Many gynecologists can and do acknowledge the limits of their expertise. They know when they have reached a point where additional knowledge is necessary. However, some have difficulty referring their patients for more specialized care. They are conflicted about letting their patients down and do not always know when to make referrals. Many hope that their patients will ask them to be referred to specialists.

Deciding to see a more qualified physician is indeed difficult for all parties. However, there are guidelines that can be helpful. Specifically, infertile patients should consult a specialist if one of the following conditions occurs:

1. if preliminary tests show no problems, yet the infertility persists for more than two years;
2. if there is a history of three or more miscarriage;
3. if the woman has irregular menstrual cycles or erratic ovulation;
4. if the man has low sperm count or motility;
5. if the woman needs treatment for endometriosis or tubal damage.[1]

* * *

If they (the couple) know there is a specialist in the area, and they are having trouble getting pregnant, it would save them time if they just go right away to a specialist. After one year of trying, then if they want to go to their gynecologist and the gynecologist wants to start a workup, fine. If you're 38 years old, it can be six months of trying. But the idea is, if you go to a busy ob/gyn practice you'll probably get "Do three months of temp charts, do three months . . . , do three months . . . ," and nobody's really looking, and taking the time to say, "Gee, she's 37, we better move fast, we don't have many years here." Where, if you're 25 years old, and you try for a year then go to your gynecologist and he does a few things, you still have a lot of time. Now that there's so much education about reproductive life, if you know enough to go to a specialist, go. Even now, some people come in and say, "I've been on Clomid a year and a half." If that's as far as they (the ob/gyn) can go, then they should be referring. But they get busy, they're human too, and they figure, "Well, she's on Clomid, we'll give her another month." And it turns into another month, unless the patient says, "Look, I've been on this a year and a half, what can we do?" And then he'll (ob/gyn) refer her when it should have been after six months. . . . They (patients) figure he knows and that's it. It's not that they don't care, it's just they never review the chart. . . . There are some ob/gyns who know they are busy with obstetrics and don't have the time to spend with infertility. Some will say, "I'll do a certain amount and if this doesn't work, I'm going to refer you."

Regina Matties R.N.

It is important to understand the difference between an infertility specialist and a board-certified specialist in reproductive endocrinology/fertility. Any gynecologist can claim to be an infertility specialist. Some may have treated women over the years for infertility problems and been successful. Their practices eventually become known as specializing in infertility. Others who believe they are specialists in the field may not have the necessary experience at all.

Endocrinology refers to the hormones and how they influence fertility. Board-certified specialists in reproductive endocrinology/fertility complete a two-year clinical fellowship besides their gynecology training. Their practice is almost solely dedicated to infertility. Most specialists will be experienced in the latest techniques and treatments.

There are many emotionally supportive advantages in going to this type of office. The doctor and staff should be very understanding of the emotional components of infertility. Furthermore, in contrast to ob/gyn offices, couples will not have to sit in a waiting room full of pregnant women and listen to all the chatter of diapers and day care. Instead, they can find comfort as they look around the specialist's waiting room and see that they are not alone.

How does one go about selecting a specialist? Usually couples first receive unsolicited referrals from friends. A friend knows a friend who got pregnant by Dr. So and So. However, this can be confusing and not necessarily the best way to obtain the name of a competent specialist. It is critical that couples separate fact from fiction, not feel obligated to any friend or relative, and choose a specialist based on solid credentials.

The more reliable source for a referral would be the woman's own gynecologist. However, because of their loyalty, many patients refer themselves. They would rather not risk offending their doctors by asking for the name of another physician. Resolve, which is a nationwide organization for infertile couples that provides support, and medical information, has compiled a *Directory of Infertility Resources.* The directory is a list of specialists across the country and can be obtained by contacting the national Resolve office. Local Resolve chapters also provide referrals.

When there are few or no specialists to choose from in the immediate area, couples have to decide how far they are willing to travel. As some procedures require frequent appointments, treatment can become time-consuming and complicated if couples travel a distance to their physicians.

> It was an hour and a half ride each way. . . . I'd have to go down there every day for blood tests and ultrasounds for about five or six days a month. I don't know how people that work on a job that can't take time off do it. I don't know how they do it. It's very demanding, you have to be there at a certain time. . . . But it was worth it to me to make the trip. I said if it's going to work I would try anything.

The Initial Consultation

It may take some time to get an appointment with a specialist, so it is important that couples not delay. During the waiting period, couples can prepare for the visit and write down any questions for the doctor. This should be done for any future appointments also.

During the initial consultation and examination, couples should evaluate both the specialist and the office staff. Couples have the right to expect that the office staff will be sensitive to their feelings and able to provide extra support when necessary. It is important that the staff are willing and able to spend time with couples, listen to their concerns, and answer questions regarding infertility and its treatment.

Especially at the first appointment, many couples feel ashamed to be at the office. Others believe this is a desperate last attempt. It is normal for couples to feel nervous and anxious before the initial appointment. However, once couples receive information, there is a sense of relief that there are practical treatment options available for their problems.

The first appointment usually involves a detailed medical history of both partners, with some questions on past contraception methods. The couple again may be intimidated by some of the personal questions, but it is important that the doctor have all pertinent information in order to make a proper diagnosis. The initial visit may also include a thorough gynecological exam. The specialist may choose to repeat some or all of the tests that were conducted by the previous physician. However, each doctor works differently.

Evaluations and Treatments

Assuming that the initial tests do not provide a reason for the infertility, additional evaluations and treatments will be planned. Some procedures may include those described in the previous chapter. However, the specialist has the ability to use more advanced techniques.

Surgical Procedures and Endometriosis

The laparoscopy, often called "belly-button" surgery or the "Band-Aid" operation, is a major step in the evaluation process. The laparoscopy is a minor diagnostic surgical procedure carried out under general anesthesia. The operation can be performed on an outpatient basis, but sometimes patients are required to stay overnight.

To begin the laparoscopy, the surgeon cuts a very small incision below the navel and one above the pubic hairline. Carbon dioxide is then pumped into the abdominal cavity so there is a clear view of the internal reproductive organs. The laparoscope, a scope with a fiber-optic light attached, is inserted and the doctor proceeds to look for endometrial tissue, adhesions, and scarring that might impede fertility. When the surgery is finished, the gas is removed from the abdomen and the incisions are bandaged.

Most doctors recommend a two- to three-day rest period after the procedure. However, research suggests that women may need one to two weeks following the laparoscopy before they regain full strength and are back to normal.[2]

There are three conditions that warrant undertaking the procedure:

1. when the etiology for the infertility is unknown despite previous tests;
2. when treatments for other problems diagnosed have not been successful;
3. when endometriosis is suspected.

Endometriosis is a disease that is found in about 20 percent of infertile women.[3] The disease involves the endometrial cells, which are normally in the lining of the uterus. In endometriosis, the endometrial cells grow outside the uterus, typically in the ovaries and abdomen. Cases range from mild to severe. Serious cases include enlarged ovaries, or even tubes blocked by large cysts and massive scar tissue. The disease does not, however, have to be directly involved with the tubes, ovaries or uterus to cause a problem. Some women do not have symptoms with a severe case, while women with a mild case experience great discomfort during their menstrual period or during intercourse. Many women feel that the diagnosis of endometriosis is ambiguous and a "rubber-stamp" diagnosis. They fear that the severity of the diagnosis can be determined by the physician's mood.

Several treatments for endometriosis are available depending on the outcome of the laparoscopy. To avoid another operation, the patient and doctor may agree before the operation that laser surgery will be performed if small amounts of endometriosis are found. If the endometriosis is significant, then other treatment will be necessary. For instance, a laparotomy, which is regular abdominal surgery, may be necessary to remove adhesions. If the surgeon finds tubal damage, perhaps microsurgical techniques, involving small-scale cutting and sewing of the tubes, may be required. Both surgeries involve a larger incision in the abdomen, an extended stay in the hospital, and an extended recovery time at home.

Another option available is drug therapy, which may be used either by itself or with surgery. The drug Danocrine is usually prescribed for endometriosis. It is derived from a male hormone and brings on a pseudomenopause to help suppress the growth of endometriosis. It has some annoying side affects such as causing weight gain, deepening of the voice, and abnormal hair growth on the face. The drug is usually taken for a period of from three to six months. This waiting period before trying to conceive again is very frustrating for most women.

With treatment, whether by drug therapy or surgery, there is still no guarantee of success. These treatments are not cures for the disease, and it can recur about 50 percent of the time.[4]

Most people find the idea of general anesthesia anxiety-producing. Many are concerned about surgical mishaps such as loss of body parts or death; others worry about how they will feel afterward. Some fear that the surgery will make the infertility worse.

> I was petrified to go through any surgery, totally petrified. The laparoscopy was the first time, and I was very sick after. I had three months of waiting for this surgery (laparotomy), it was the worst three months of my life. It was just awful. My biggest fear was going under the anesthesia. Not for what they were going to find or do, but I think for the anesthesia alone.

For some women, the laparoscopy may be their first surgical experience, and their anticipatory anxiety can manifest itself in the form of sleepless nights, crying and irritability. Making specific preparations with the spouse and/or other significant persons for additional support will cause the procedure to be more tolerable. In addition, many women want as much preparative information as they can get, so that they know exactly what is going to be done.

The laparoscopy can be a major step in the life crisis of an infertile person. As with any surgery, there is a tremendous range of emotions experienced. Some women may feel relief and renewal, while others feel depression and resignation. Women who are infertile are often angry that the surgery is required. Some women will feel very proud of themselves for having gone through it. Even so, the surgery will usually change most women in some way. The scars that remain can be a reminder of being "damaged and malfunctioning."

Many women place unrealistically high hopes on the procedure and expect the laparoscopy to be a sufficient curative. If that is not to be, they hope the doctor will find a treatable problem. When no problems are discovered, women experience mixed emotions. There is a sense of relief with the knowledge that everything is all right. However, sadness is also felt as the cause of the infertility continues to allude them.

Pergonal

Pergonal, or human menopausal gonadotropin, (HMG) is another treatment for infertility. Pergonal is a natural hormone that bypasses the brain and acts directly on the ovaries. It is used when Clomid has failed. Although Pergonal is becoming more commonplace, patients cannot underestimate its strength.

Pergonal has some side effects that need to be considered by couples before beginning treatment. One major concern is multiple births. Twenty percent of births from Pergonal will be more than one baby, with twins being most common.[5] With proper monitoring, the quintuplets that are brought to the public's attention by the tabloids can be avoided. Another risk of Pergonal therapy is hyperstimulation of the ovaries. In some cases, the ovaries have enlarged to the size of a basketball, resulting in serious medical complications. Proper monitoring reduces the risks associated with hyperstimulation. With side effects being so severe, couples should receive Pergonal only from a physician who has extensive experience with the treatment.

Pergonal treatment is expensive, about $1000 to $1500 per cycle, and very demanding. The procedure involves a series of five to ten injections of HMG, one to four injections of HCG, several blood tests to monitor the levels of estrogen and progesterone, and several ultrasounds to monitor the development of the follicles. It is no wonder that a woman can feel like a pin cushion after a single cycle of Pergonal.

After couples have decided to undergo Pergonal treatment, women need to choose a method for receiving the intramuscular injections. Some women choose to administer the medication themselves. Others are more comfortable if a professional gives the injection. Thus, they look for a friend with a nursing background. However, the majority have the medication given to them by their husbands, after training by the physician's staff. Some of the men are nervous, but willing to do their part. Women also feel some trepidation about having their husbands give them daily injections. In the end, couples benefit because the treatment takes place in the comfort and privacy of their homes.

> I was very nervous at first, and actually surprised he agreed to do it. I never thought my husband would be able to give me the shots. He's this 6'2", 200 lb. jock with big hands. But I was pleasantly surprised, he was gentler than the nurses! And what's nice about it, afterwards you get a big hug. Something the nurses don't do.

To maximize the chances for pregnancy, many specialists also incorporate a procedure called intrauterine insemination (IUI) with Pergonal therapy. IUI is a form of artificial insemination that uses the husband's sperm. In IUI, the semen specimen undergoes a procedure called sperm-washing to remove all impurities. Several hours later, the sperm is injected into the uterine cavity directly through the cervical canal. The procedure is simple. However, some couples are offended when they think about the impersonal, sterile nature of this reproductive process.

The Pergonal regimen can be emotionally draining as well. Aside from the almost daily injections and constant trips to the specialist's office, the associated feelings are intense. When couples are approached with the suggestion of Pergonal, they are often shocked. Pergonal has always been thought of as the drug for women with "real" problems. Many feel that it is their last resort short of in vitro fertilization, and for those who cannot afford IVF, it may be. Others place too much faith in the drug. They think that if it can produce five or six babies for some, surely it can give them at least one or two.

> On some of my Pergonal cycles I was producing as many as four follicles. I thought to myself, "At least one of these four should take." I couldn't believe it. I was really hoping for twins so I'd be finished with all of this. But nothing ever happened.

Pergonal has about a 50 percent conception rate.[6] With the high hopes for a pregnancy, many couples also express a desire to have twins and "get it over with." However, after eight, ten, or twelve cycles on Pergonal many hopes come crashing down. For these couples, Pergonal is not the wonder drug they had envisioned it to be, and another decision must be made.

In Vitro Fertilization

The major breakthrough in the last decade in infertility treatment has been in vitro fertilization (IVF) and other related procedures such as gamete intrafallopian tube transfer (GIFT) and zygote intrafallopian tube transfer (ZIFT). There are currently about two hundred clinics in the United States that do in vitro fertilization, with some clinics having more experience than others.[7]

In IVF, the eggs are fertilized outside the body, then transferred back to the uterus to develop. With GIFT, the sperm and egg are mixed and injected into the Fallopian tube, allowing normal fertilization and implantation to occur. ZIFT is similar to IVF because the eggs are fertilized outside the body. However, like GIFT, the zygote is injected into the Fallopian tube.

Originally, IVF was intended for women with blocked or damaged tubes. Now it is offered to those patients with immunologic or unexplained infertility and those who have had repeated ectopic pregnancies. It also may be helpful for some male infertility problems such as low sperm count and poor motility.

In all three procedures, the process begins by stimulating follicle development with Pergonal or Clomid. Careful monitoring follows, using ultrasound and blood tests, to determine when an adequate number of follicles have developed. At the appropriate time, the eggs are retrieved either by laparoscopy or ultrasound-guided aspiration techniques. A semen sample is obtained and the sperm-washing procedure is used in preparation for fertilization.

In the IVF procedure, the sperm is then mixed in a culture dish with as many as nine eggs. Next, the culture is incubated for almost forty-eight hours under highly controlled conditions. The specimen is closely monitored to determine whether fertilization and cell division occur. When or if the zygote reaches the eight-cell stage, it is transferred to the uterus via a catheter and syringe in hopes that it implants. After transfer, women remain in bed from one to twelve hours and then wait another two weeks for the pregnancy test results.

In theory, the procedures sound simple, but there are few guarantees. It is a very demanding process, and anything can go wrong along the way.

The success rates for IVF are between 10 and 20 percent.[8] Failures fall into the following categories:

> 20 percent of patients have inadequate follicular maturation;
> 15 percent fail to implant;
> 25 to 30 percent spontaneously abort before the first missed period;
> 10 percent miscarry later.[9]

Initially, IVF clinics screen their patients to ensure that they have exhausted others means of treatment. There are other qualifying variables as well. Age is usually a factor. Some clinics will not accept women older than thirty-five years of age. Money is another consideration. IVF costs between $5000 and $8000 per cycle. Couples can expect to undergo at least three to four cycles at a minimum. If travel to the clinic is necessary, lost work time and the cost of accommodations are additional burdens.

Each step of the treatment is grueling for couples. They are constantly anxious. They worry about how many follicles will develop, if the doctor will be able to retrieve the eggs, if they will implant, and so on. They know that at any time the whole process can end. IVF has been described as a "final exam that I prayed to pass." Finally, many clinics limit the number of IVF attempts to three or four, even when the couple is emotionally and financially stable. Again there is that deadline that must be met.

Many couples are not realistic about the low probability of pregnancy with IVF. Even though most couples are well-informed about the procedure itself, many choose not to believe the low success rates. They believe IVF is their "last resort," or the "end of the road." Although some will apply for adoption, even during the process, most couples who choose IVF have "staked all hopes and dreams on it."

Some clinics employ counselors to interview couples before undergoing IVF. Few clinics offer continuing counseling or psychological support. Counselors working with IVF patients attempt to help the couples realistically evaluate their chances of having a child through IVF. However, even when couples state they understand their odds of success, they are not always honest. For some, IVF becomes an obsession.

Studies show that when an attempt with IVF fails, women will experience a grief reaction similar to that associated with pregnancy loss.[10] When undergoing the procedure, patients have often developed strong attachment to the fertilized eggs, thinking of the eggs as strong, viable babies. As one woman puts it, "I never expected to bond so much with embryos." When the process fails to produce a pregnancy, some women go beyond the normal limits of sadness and disappointment. They become extremely depressed, with varying degrees of hostility and guilt.[11] The intensity of these feelings is the greatest after the first cycle.

Some women express the feeling of being alone during the IVF process and complain about the lack of personal contact with the physician. Other patients seem to bond with one another.[12] Some will seek the support of friends and family; others do not want their friends and relatives "to follow this thing with me on a daily basis." With or without support, each step is emotionally intense.

On a positive note, men are not as prone to the same strong emotional reactions as are their spouses. Thus, they are psychologically able to be supportive.[13]

Kathleen and Daniel have been through five in vitro fertilization attempts. For one cycle, Kathleen produced only two follicles and the doctors did not feel that retrieval was warranted. For two additional cycles, she produced seven follicles. The doctors retrieved the seven follicles at each cycle, but on both occasions, none fertilized. For the other two cycles Kathleen and Daniel reached the transfer stage. Once, three follicles were produced and two fertilized. The other cycle produced nine follicles and four fertilized. However, none of the zygotes implanted.

Daniel

If they cancel a cycle after I've been injecting her for three to five days, or eight days, that's depressing. You're always saying, "I wished they could have at least gone to retrieval, to get the eggs out."But if they went for retrieval, and the eggs took and then went for implant, then you wait around for two weeks and find out they didn't implant, that's really depressing.

Kathleen

For me, it was worse when we'd go for retrieval. I'm not crazy about the epidurals—the last one was horrible. It was worse when we went for retrieval, got the seven eggs, and wound up with nothing. I would rather have them cancel a cycle than go through retrieval and come up empty. That to me was harder. Once they get the eggs, then you have to wait for them to call and tell you how many fertilized. Then they tell you nothing happened . . . I wanted to kill somebody.

Daniel

They're all nice people there. When we'd go for retrieval everyone would be happy and there's a lot of talking. Everyone's so friendly that it intensifies your depression in the end. Everyone's saying, "We're sure this is going to be the one." It boosts you up more. If it was a little more "sterile," you wouldn't get so excited.

The Emotions of Extended Infertility

In the beginning stages of infertility, couples confront a wide range of emotions, sometimes for the first time. As infertility persists, the frequency and intensity of these emotions increase. To some, the emotions seem unbearable, as the affect can be more intense than anything previously experienced. People may believe they are losing their minds and headed for an emotional breakdown. Psychiatric symptoms may appear.

Anger predominates as individuals develop short fuses and their patience with others diminishes. We often can accept expressions of anger in moderate doses. For infertile couples, the anger borders on rage. Anger is directed toward themselves, their spouses, their families, and their God. Often the anger is directed at the seeming unfairness of others' unwanted fertility. Parents who abuse or abandon a child, the person who has an elected abortion, and the relative with a surprise pregnancy all become targets for the anger. The anger creates considerable discomfort for others because people are not usually exposed to this degree of rage in the normal course of events.

The inability to reproduce strikes at the core of human essence. Hopes, dreams, and goals that have been nurtured from youth are at risk of being shattered. Infertility invades human sexuality and seriously injures self-esteem. Couples are no longer able to control significant aspects of their lives. They are left with a sense of emptiness, one that they fear they will never be able to fill. As the treatment persists, there is a pessimistic belief by couples that all the past dreams were in vain and major adjustments will need to be made in life plans. As feelings of loss develop into depression and despair, many people who are infertile become prone to crying at the least opportune moments.

> His friend Joe called Christmas Eve in between churches. So that kind of set us off. We were thinking about it (the miscarriage) but the call brought everything back. Joe was very upset about his wife's miscarriage, it brought everything home. Church was very difficult. I had a real hard time in church. The priest opened his mouth and I started crying I have no idea why. And I'm not even Catholic! It was Bill's (husband) church. . . . I don't particularly feel emotional in church. I don't know what set me off. It wasn't anything I could control. It overwhelmed me, which surprised me. . . . I couldn't control it. Usually if it's just a little bit I can say, "Come on, let's get ourselves together and get through this. You can cry in the car." But I couldn't wait. I'm going to do it now. I'm going to cry all I want. It's the weirdest feeling. I never expected to lose it in church.

As infertility persists and changes into a chronic condition, stress and anxiety intensify. What started as an inconvenience to be dealt with has turned into a life crisis of major significance. With the exposure to the continual stress, forgetfulness increases and persons appear less organized. At this point, coping becomes hard work.

Hans Seyle developed the general adaptation syndrome to describe reactions to chronic stress.[14] It is applicable to people dealing with prolonged infertility. In the Seyle's model, there are three stages of reaction. In the first stage, which is labeled alarm, anxiety, fear, depression, and mental disorganization disrupt the total level of functioning. As the stressor continues, we adapt to the stress because a level of resistance builds. Hence, the second stage is the resistance stage. If the stresses persist, couples confront the third stage, exhaustion. Coping mechanisms break down and emotional and physical reactions become more intense, with hopelessness and apathy evident. In this stage, coping becomes strained and affects other areas of life including work, family, and other social relationships.

Ambiguity also plays a significant role in the emotional responses of the infertile. Although it is known that 5 percent of infertile couples are diagnosed as "cause unknown," many go for extended periods of time without knowing the reasons for the infertility. This ambiguity increases anxiety, making the lack of control more difficult to handle.[15]

> They still, to this day, cannot give me a reason why it didn't work. It's frustrating. You want somebody to give you some explanation, anybody, anything. Just tell me why. Sometimes I feel it's harder if you don't have a reason. You feel like you want somebody or something to blame, or somebody you can at least take out your anger and frustration on. And there's nothing. Nobody can give you any answer. It's hard.

As any infertile person knows, there are certain events that are very painful. Christmas holidays, baby showers, christenings, and children's birthday parties, are just some of the events that cause the infertile to experience all the negative emotions they so strongly associate with their infertility. Sometimes the anticipatory anxiety related to these events can cause sleeplessness and an unbearable tension for days prior to the event.

> Christmas was thrown together. If my parents hadn't been coming, we both discussed that we would not have had any decorations. We worked on the cellar because we had to get it ready for my parents—that's not why we were working on the cellar. It was so we would be working until 11 o'clock at night and drowning ourselves in this, and not have to deal with holidays coming up. If my parents weren't coming we probably wouldn't have put up the decorations. The tree went up last minute, and we were still putting up decorations Christmas Eve. We didn't have any desire to do it. I'm surprised it affected me that much. We didn't go to

one Christmas party this year, we ignored it all. I just couldn't fake it. No celebration of the holidays at all. It's amazing. I didn't expect that, not to the point that we had to cancel things because I couldn't deal with it. I was real surprised about that.

Couples continually cope with infertility until they achieve some degree of resolution. Some couples are more successful than others. To reduce the pain and distress related to infertility, couples who achieve a level of acceptance realize they have little control over the achievement of pregnancy. However, this level of acceptance does not come easily. In Menning's model of infertility, the resolution stage comes after an extended period of considerable distress and pain.[16] Even then, resolution does not necessarily mean that all the emotions of the past have been put behind one. There is a degree of acceptance of the infertility and the emotions that developed out of it. The depression and anger do not disappear, they become less debilitating and easier to manage.

Counseling Strategies

Most counselors should feel they have the ability to work successfully with infertile couples. Training programs in social work, counseling, and psychology teach the basic counseling skills that are most important when working with couples who are distressed by their infertility. Couples who are infertile need support, warmth and acceptance to assist them with the overwhelming feelings they are experiencing. Decision making may also be a focus of counseling. As counselors have these skills in their repertoires, it is not necessary to discuss their use in detail. However, because of the dynamics of infertility, there are some special strategies that couples will find useful to help them cope. Counselors, clergy, and other helping professionals should be aware of these strategies so they can use them when appropriate.

Take Control Where Possible

Coping is made difficult by the lack of control experienced when couples struggle with infertility. We are reared in a society that believes that people can attain almost anything they want if they work hard. With infertility, such a belief system is contradicted and problematic. Working hard will not solve the infertility. In fact, many fertile people believe the myth that infertility is caused by trying too hard. Thus, many people tell the infertile couple to relax and not to try so hard. Henceforth, couples respond by working hard to relax. These attempts are futile as anxiety continues with each unsuccessful month. Such is the bind of the infertile couple.

Couples need to realize that their inability to achieve pregnancy is but one part of their lives. They may not be able to control their fertility. However, they can control other aspects such as whether they go on vacation, search for a different job, or move to a new location. Couples need to make decisions about those other areas of their lives when appropriate. Couples can identify those other areas that contribute to their unhappiness. They should be encouraged to deal with those issues. Career choices, vacation plans, housing purchases, should not be put off with the idea that pregnancy will happen soon. The more couples' decisions are made based on plans for a child, the greater will be the anger when pregnancy does not occur.

Take Charge of Treatment

For the couple's mental health, they should regain as much control as possible over their lives. Although couples cannot regulate conception, they can control other aspects of their infertility treatment. As infertility persists, it is important to maximize the perception that the couple is in charge of their own lives. One way to do this is by involving them in the treatment regime.

Although treatment takes place under the supervision of the physician, couples need to be active members of the treatment team. By discussing possible strategies that they may have read about, or questioning the known effectiveness of certain treatments, couples can be assertive in their role of developing a realistic treatment plan with the physician. This plan can be flexible and subject to change based on discussion with the physician. It would simply be a road map, one over which the couple would have direct input and control.

At my twelve month appointment (being on Clomid) I pretty much laid into the doctor and said, "No, nothing's happening, let's get going." He was basically saying, "We'll try different things, and we've been trying different things. It's just a matter of getting the right recipe for your body." I went in one time fuming mad. Within seconds anything I wanted to discuss, or argue about, or say there's a problem about, was all gone. He just had that way of calming you down, and everything you wanted to discuss or was angry about, went out the window. It was very frustrating for me. I still kept saying to myself, "That's OK, you're going to have your chance, you're going to have your chance." Then he starts talking about the future plans and this next cycle. He says, "This is what we're going to do." He planned it all out. I said, "OK, now's my chance." And he gets up and leaves the room to write the prescriptions. . . . I was probably more angry with myself. I'm not one of those people who can say, "Wait a minute, I want to talk, it's my turn." I just can't put my foot down.

An important aspect of a treatment plan is treatment holidays. The struggle to conceive is ongoing and puts enormous amounts of stress on the couple. Taking a holiday allows the couple to enjoy the time without pressure to have sex, or to wonder, as day 28 approaches, whether this will be the month. Treatment holidays may be critical for maintaining the mental health of the couple.

The most relaxed times during our eight years of treatment were the months when pregnancy was not possible. Initially, they were forced onto us because of miscarriage, or a specific treatment which required medication for several months. Later, we made conscious decisions to take a month off. At first we thought we wasted those months. However, we were eventually able to realize, how much easier those times were when we were not trying to have a baby.

Develop Purposeful Positive Experiences

Infertility, with its treatment, is a very emotionally punishing experience with many highs and lows. Couples feel disappointment, anger, and despair when menstruation appears, followed by periods of renewed hope and optimism when the cycle begins again. To help counter the emotional exhaustion that occurs, couples need to be very active in planning positive experiences for themselves. A vacation might be taken around the planned treatment holiday. If money has been saved for future child-oriented expenses, they may want to take some of it for a more lavish trip.

People need to reward themselves when they have been successful in any area of their lives. Although this advice is appropriate for any individual, it is most important for the mental health of the infertile. The loss of self-esteem can be such that they forget they are worthy people who have a wide range of strengths and competencies.

In addition, if one or both have undergone an especially painful procedure, it is appropriate that they treat themselves to something special. Many things can be done within any budget. Some rewards would include a special meal, a weekend away, a night out on the town. The activities should be positive and pleasurable and provide a break from the negative feelings associated with the infertility. Couples need to understand the importance of taking care of themselves during this stressful period of their lives.

Plan Coping Strategies

When an individual or couple believe a certain event would cause too much pain, then avoiding the event would be an appropriate alternative. Planned avoiding is important for maintaining mental health and should be practiced when necessary without guilt. Although it might be easier to make up an excuse about not attending, it would be appropriate to say something like, "I am not attending the shower because it would be too difficult for me. Please give everyone my best. I am sure they understand." No one can be expected constantly to deal with infertility's depth of emotions. Friends and relatives need to understand that self preservation is critical in coping with infertility.

> Everyone thought we were away at the cabin for Thanksgiving, but we stayed home. . . . We were putting us first. We decided a while ago that it didn't matter what our families thought about us at this point. It was survival on our part. We were very selfish. We weren't even attempting to be human people, we wanted to be

alone and that was the way it was going to be. . . . We made a conscious effort to be with each other and do what we wanted to do.

If the couple decides to attend a certain event, even if they expect it to be stressful, there are some things they can do to help themselves. They can plan, and even rehearse, how they will cope while they are there. For example, if they expect that being with family at the holidays will bring to the surface feelings that one or both would prefer not to deal with, then the couple might plan to leave after a short period of time. Furthermore, they might develop signals for each other if they feel they are losing control and they would want assistance or additional support. Avoiding discussions that would bring up the unwanted feelings is also possible. Whatever, the more time couples spend talking about how they want to handle the event, the better they will feel going into the event. At last, they should prepare for the unexpected emotional expressions that might occur and rehearse how they will handle them. At this point it is important that they understand that the feelings they are experiencing are typical of infertility. Crying or outbursts of anger will occur, especially when they least want them to. Thus, the couple needs to support each other in the expression of their emotions when with others.

The final planned task is based on recent psychological advances. There is a school of thought in psychology led by Albert Ellis and Donald Meichenbaum, among others, that believes our thought processes are controlled by our emotions.[17,18] Thus, if we are experiencing negative emotions, it is because we are having thoughts that are bringing these emotions to the surface. The key to changing how we feel is to change how we think. Infertile couples can moderate some of their emotional experiences by changing their thought patterns. Some examples that show the differences between negative and positive thinking are given below.

Negatives	*Positive Alternatives*
I need a child to be fulfilled.	I would like to have a child very much. However, I do not need a child to be fulfilled.

Negatives	Positive Alternatives
	There are many aspects of my life that bring fulfillment.
I will be devastated if this treatment doesn't work.	I will be upset if this treatment fails. However, I will handle it just as I have handled the other disappointments.
I will let my spouse and my family down if I can't have a child.	I understand that others feel bad that we do not have children. However, I am not responsible for how others feel. I am doing what I can and I hope they accept that.
I will never be able to handle it if the doctor tells me I can't have children.	I will be able to cope with anything the doctor tells me. I may be upset and disappointed, but I will survive.

Spouses can help support each other's positive statements. Again, these require that couples work hard at coping. They may not make the feelings go away entirely—nothing does; they only make them manageable.

Relaxation Strategies

Despite what well-meaning friends and relatives say, relaxing will not help achieve pregnancy. However, it will help couples cope. As a chronic condition, infertility can be physically and mentally wearing. The anxiety makes sleep that much harder, thus increasing the anxiety and contributing to a cycle that has many additional negative effects. To combat this cycle, there are some things that can be done to assist in alleviating the anxiety, reducing the tensions, and increasing the overall sense of well-being. These things would all come under the heading of relaxation exercises.

One of the simplest ways of relaxing is exercise. Any regular regimen of exercise should be under a doctor's supervision. With infertile women, this is especially true as rigorous exercise such as jogging can affect the menstrual cycle. Weight loss could also impede fertility. With these cautions in mind, exercise does provide an opportunity to engage in something positive while providing a distraction from the infertility. With competitive sports, such as tennis or basketball, the forced concentration almost mandates that the participant focus on the game at hand, thus leaving little room for thinking about other issues. The second benefit of exercise is that, when completed, participants feel relaxed accompanied by a positive sense of accomplishment. Sleep is also likely to come more easily.

Progressive muscle relaxation is another way to manage stress while increasing your sense of positive well-being. With muscle relaxation, the subject takes charge of felt anxiety by systematically tightening and then relaxing all muscle groups. Also, care is taken to breathe deliberately, slowly, and deeply. There are commercial tapes available that direct subjects through the sequence. However, specific sequences are available in other published forms and can be easily learned. The entire process can be completed in thirty minutes. It is important that the time involved is free from distractions.

Meditation is another way to increase a feeling of well-being. Meditation was popular in the sixties and early seventies when many young people were trying to find themselves. Transcendental meditation was widely known at the time.

In meditation, the subject focuses thoughts and energy onto one idea. There are many similarities to the progressive muscle relaxation. The subject sits in a comfortable position, breathing is slow, deep, and deliberate, and the person spends about twenty uninterrupted minutes meditating. Meditation is more of a mental exercise as compared with progressive relaxation's physical emphasis. In meditation, all else is forgotten as the subject attempts to maintain a blank mind. Relaxation comes at its own pace.

Finally, the martial arts provide a way of combining the three techniques. The martial arts are based on many of the same philosophical roots as meditation. With both, there is an emphasis on self-control, especially in terms of thought processes. In addition, a vigorous martial arts program contains a high degree of physical exercise. Some, especially karate and judo, contain exercises that involve the systematic process of tensing and relaxing muscles.

Support Networks

Many people who are infertile feel unworthy, different, and alone. Comments made to them by people who have not experienced infertility reinforce this belief system. As a result, people who are infertile withdraw from others. Although they isolate themselves to avoid the unpleasant feelings, the result is that they eventually feel more alone and different. It can be a difficult bind.

Counseling groups and social support networks consisting of other couples who are infertile can be most useful, especially for those couples who are feeling particularly isolated. These groups provide people who are infertile an opportunity to meet others and to talk and listen about their infertility. Although couples may be initially hesitant to join a group, these couples eventually come to understand what research had demonstrated long ago:[19] these groups increase participants' sense of hope and help them develop a sense of belonging. In addition, they increase the members' sense of control by providing resources and information about infertility. Finally, by listening to others who have successfully coped with their infertility, other couples who are infertile hear strategies that may be useful in their own struggle.

Barbara Eck Menning understood infertile couples' needs for sharing their feelings and for listening to how others are coping with their problems. As a result, she founded Resolve, Inc., a support organization for people who are infertile managed by others who are infertile. Since its inception in 1973, Resolve has grown into a large national organization committed to providing information and support to infertile couples. In addition, other support groups for infertility, endometriosis, and pregnancy loss have been organized throughout the country. Besides the formal support group, these organizations typically sponsor seminars and informal discussions that explore problems with achieving pregnancy. Helpers should encourage infertile couples to take advantage of these programs.

The Positive Side of Infertility

For the Chinese, crisis is represented by two symbols, danger and opportunity. The dangers of infertility are well documented and account for the major part of any discussion involving infertility. However, the opportunities should not be left out. Infertility is a major crisis for most who face it. It may be the first crisis couples have faced together, the most difficult one, and one that they initially believed they could never successfully endure. As time progresses, they realize they have endured the crisis. They have survived, and maybe learned some new things about themselves. They can develop a sense of personal accomplishment, one that can enhance self-esteem. For the couples, infertility stresses the marital relationship, but, with understanding and determination, the marriage can be stronger and more fulfilling than before. In the end, infertility can have some positive benefits. Counselors can assist couples find the positive in the experience. They can help couples maintain a sense of hope when the situation looks its worst. Counselors can reassure couples that they have the strength and resources to overcome the obstacles. Finally, counselors, clergy, and other helpers can assist couples who are infertile identify the positive outcomes from the infertility experience. For us, our infertility allowed us to demonstrate a personal strength we never thought existed. The infertility experiences also challenged our marriage but brought us closer as a couple and thus made our marriage stronger. Finally, the experience brought us the best thing we will have ever known. We will describe that benefit more fully in the last chapter.

6

Marital Issues

Without children, a marriage is merely a legal compact in which both partners look to each other for protection and shelter, a very sensible arrangement for all those who would just as soon not leave their emotional and sexual needs to the chancy business of meeting the right person for the night in a swinging bar, and who, if they pool their belongings and their hopes, would very sensibly like to have something in writing to confirm the arrangement.[1]

For most, children are an important and expected outcome of marriage. Ninety five percent of couples begin their marital relationships with the expectation that they will someday have children.[2] As previously indicated, 20 percent will eventually face the possibility that they may not have children, at least in the way they originally believed it would happen. For them, infertility is indeed a crisis in the marriage.

Previously, we have delineated the dynamics of infertility, especially as it affects individuals. Treatment as well as psychological issues for both women and men were discussed, and coping strategies were suggested. However, the degree to which individuals successfully deal with their own issues of infertility is intrinsically related to the marital system's ability to handle the stress.

The roller coaster of emotions experienced during the struggle will turn marriages upside down and inside out. Infertility will pull the marriage in several directions at once, resulting in either the deterioration or strengthening of the relationship.

Research, although equivocal, shows that both happen. For

94

instance, Berger studied the relationship of sixteen couples who attended a reproduction biology clinic in a general hospital. The couples were interviewed after the men were found to be infertile. Within the sixteen couples, ten men had problems of impotence within one week of the diagnosis. One man and three women had affairs. Finally, six of the sixteen women were significantly more angry at their husbands after the diagnosis.[3]

Research also indicates that struggling with infertility can result in strong marital bonds. As an example, fifty eight couples attending the Jones Institute of Reproductive Medicine reported only a minimal amount of marital dysfunction, with the majority reporting a strong husband-wife relationship.[4]

Indeed, infertility can make some marriages less stable, especially those that were dysfunctional before the diagnosis. Usually the degree of instability is associated with the duration of the infertility. The longer infertility persists, the greater the stress on the marriage and, as a result, the greater the negative effect infertility has on the marital system.

At the same time, infertility can strengthen some marital bonds. This usually happens among those couples who realize they are not alone in their infertility—that it is common to many couples. Those positive changes are associated with overcoming a life crisis together. Thus, couples who overcome the stress of infertility and make the decision to go to a clinic that specializes in in vitro fertilization, such as the Jones's clinic, show the ways in which infertility can strengthen a marriage.

When couples are told that they are infertile, they experience predictable feelings and problems. As briefly discussed in Chapter 3, Barbara Eck Menning described the feelings as occurring in a series of stages. Each partner may go through the stages at a different pace. One partner may get stuck in one stage for an extended period of time. Indeed, the degree to which couples can deal with each other's feelings, both those that differ and those that are similar, will determine how well the relationship will survive the problems that occur.

In this chapter, we will explore the feelings and dynamics associated with Menning's first four stages of infertility (the last three will be discussed in the final two chapters).[5] In addition, we will discuss two areas, sexuality and communication, that are important parts of couples' experiences with infertility. Counselors, clergy, and other helping professionals have the task of assisting couples progress through the stages.

Surprise

Initially, most couples are surprised that they experience problems with conceiving. In the early stages of marital relationships, many couples worry about becoming pregnant and use contraceptives to prevent an unwanted pregnancy. The concern then shifts to choosing the right time to begin having a family. Rarely is there discussion about the possibility of being infertile. Some may not expect pregnancy to happen immediately because either the woman's mother had problems conceiving, the woman has irregular periods, or because they have friends with problems. However, couples do expect conception to eventually occur.

Denial

Research suggests that couples are most stressed during the initial consultation.[6] They cannot understand why their bodies are not cooperating. When the diagnosis of infertility, their worst fear, is realized, the flood of emotions can be overwhelming. Thus, couples need a way to cope with these new emotions until they can better understand the reality of infertility. Many couples need to absorb the diagnosis of infertility at their own pace. Denying the existence of their condition allows couples this time.

Sigmund Freud initially conceptualized defense mechanisms as ways people control anxiety resulting from external and internal threats.[7] Denial is one such defense mechanism. Denial works by maintaining the status quo until the person feels able to handle the threat. Infertility presents such a threat, distorting people's sense of self, ruining dreams, and altering the stability of marital systems. Understandably, couples need time to prepare for the threat.

Denial can take many forms. Couples may pretend the problem doesn't exist. Many couples go doctor-shopping, seeking third and fourth opinions, hoping they will find someone to tell them everything is all right. Others will not follow through with the workup. Some may hear the diagnosis, but will minimize its importance. They may believe the tests are inconclusive; or change their minds about the importance of conception. They believe they are not ready for children at this time and that their difficulty is for the better. In short, they refuse to come to terms with infertility.

In many instances, friends and family help to support the denial by telling couples just to relax and let pregnancy happen. Even physicians help couples avoid the inevitable. There are too many stories of gynecologists telling women who have unsuccessfully attempted pregnancy for one or more years to "go on a vacation";"take a bottle of wine and have a good time"; "don't worry about it yet." However, eventually reality does creep in. Thus, other emotions begin to surface as couples' struggles begin.

Isolation

When the denial no longer works, infertile couples begin to notice that everyone else is having children except them. While they are failing at conception, every friend, sister, or work mate seems to be achieving pregnancy rather easily. The emotions can be overwhelming. Therefore, to maintain emotional stability, infertile couples begin to isolate themselves from those groups of people that make them uncomfortable. Couples cope with infertility at this stage by withdrawing from the fertile world.

Infertile couples learn to gracefully decline invitations to events that are particularly stressful. Children's birthday parties, Mother's and Father's Day picnics, christenings, and brisses are among the gatherings they avoid. Couples prefer to stay away from these events so they will not have to deal with the intense feelings that they fear will surface. For women, baby showers are particularly hard. All the attention given to the mother-to-be, and seeing all the baby gifts can make for a difficult time.

Christmas or Chanuka is especially stressful for most infertile couples. The holiday season centers around children and represents so much of what couples desire. New Years and the related celebrations also serve as a milestone—that it has been one more year without a baby.

Some couples will go through the motions of the holiday, decorating a tree and buying the necessary gifts. However, the absence of toys under the tree can be too much to bear as couples are reminded of their childlessness everywhere. Others will get through the holidays by, again, declining those certain invitations that make them feel uncomfortable. Still others may opt to totally isolate themselves from family and relatives. Instead, they choose to have a private holiday celebration that avoids all the painful reminders of their infertility.

> When Christmas came, to be honest, I had no use for it whatsoever. Usually, I'm one of those people who enjoys Christmas a great deal. I enjoy getting presents for people. But I had no use for it. I didn't want to decorate. . . . The Christmas tree went up Christmas Eve just because I felt I was required to do it. And it came down two days after Christmas.

Additional problems occur when couples isolate themselves from the very same people who may give them the support they need. As a result, many try to maintain old relationships but are not always successful. However, sometimes it is better to avoid friends and uncomfortable situations than to deal with the intense feelings. It is an impossible choice.

> Sue's baby sometimes bothers me. We were over the other night and they said, "Gee, now that you're here, why don't you help us put the crib together?" Which was nice (sarcastic) right after the miscarriage. We hadn't avoided them, and I'm sure she didn't expect us to react this way, me anyhow. The crib just set us off. We wanted to get out of there real soon. It was hard to get out of the situation. . . . We weren't thinking of ourselves at the time, but more of how we should act socially. We shouldn't have done that. We should have said, "This is how it is, we've got to go." I think they thought they were trying to help by doing this.

Infertile couples give high priority to their problem. Much of their time, energy, and money are spent in pursuit of a baby.

Because others do not share this value, couples' isolation from friends, family, and relatives intensifies.

Initially, couples usually do not have enough information about their particular problem. Once they find out where to get the information, they spend their free time reading articles and books pertaining to infertility. In addition, considerable amounts of time may be spent at the doctor's office, especially with more involved therapies such as Pergonal. These couples are at the mercy of blood tests and ultrasounds that at times require daily office visits. If they are missing too much work because of treatment, they may have to make that time up. Some may have to work two jobs in order to pay for the procedures. Friendships can become secondary to the goal of conceiving a child.

Couples also deal with infertility by withdrawing from each other. Wives feel their husbands do not understand the importance of pregnancy and of having a baby. Men may believe their presence only upsets their wives. As a result, they avoid their wives whenever possible. At the least, they avoid conversations about each other's feelings.

> I got to the point where I didn't even want to talk to him about it. If I wanted to talk about adoption or something, then he didn't want to talk about it. I felt like he didn't really want to have kids anyway, and I resented it a lot. I couldn't get through to him why it was important to me. I still sometimes wonder. It's hard for me sometimes to figure out why it's so important. It's not like I figure that's a woman's purpose in life, because I don't. It's just something I've always wanted. It's one of the only things I really wanted that badly. . . . I really wanted to try in vitro. I didn't care what it cost. But he didn't want to talk about anything for awhile. I thought that he thought I'd forget about it.

> Men look at it (trying to conceive) as a big expense. It's not as emotional to them, I think, until after they see their child. . . . Before you have the baby they just think of it as a big expense. It's like one big responsibility and a lot of money down the drain, which is how I figured he looked at it.

> I said to him, "How would you feel if somebody told you that you're never going to make any more money than you are today? You're never going to have any more than you have right now." Take away all their dreams, all their goals, all the things that they

want. It's the only way to get him to understand how important it is to me.

Couples question each other's motives. Wives wonder if their husbands truly want children because they seem disinterested in sex. Husbands, however, feel rejected because they think that their wives only desire sexual intercourse in order to conceive babies. Furthermore, because of the resulting withdrawal, they do not have the opportunities to discuss their feelings. As a result, the isolation and withdrawal can become parts of a destructive cycle.

> We've been through several failed pregnancies and each time she would get depressed and I'd be a little more left out because she'd say, "I didn't care, I didn't feel anything."
> The biggest thing that bothers me is that a little over two years ago, before we even started IVF, she started sleeping on the couch. I don't know why, I'm afraid to approach her about it. . . . It started out innocently, she'd fall asleep while she was watching TV. But I always thought there was something more to it, like the more she tried to have kids and couldn't, the more she was just ignoring me. She says when we have a kid she'll come back and sleep in the bedroom.
> At one point, when we were just going to start the IVF program, she told me if I wasn't interested in having a kid I could leave now.

Anger

The denial and isolation result because couples want to avoid their own feelings. However, the avoided becomes inevitable and feelings surface. Anger is one of the strongest feelings to emerge.

For couples, infertility is a series of uncomfortable, sometimes painful experiences. There are

> doctors appointments, too numerous to count;
> rushed internal exams;
> masturbating into jars;
> their sexual relationship under constant monitoring;

insensitive friends and relatives;
failed dreams;
postcoital examinations;
unsuccessful treatments;
missed sexual opportunities resulting in a wasted month;
delayed career opportunities;
pregnancy at last, followed by a miscarriage;
missed family affairs;
a poorly planned business trip resulting in another wasted
    month;
another pregnant friend;
menstruation one week late;
medication side effects;
doctor's office vacations resulting in another wasted month;
surgery;
many wasted months turned into years.

As couples face more events from the list, the stress and strain can become unbearable. No matter how successful couples are at isolating themselves from hurtful others, painful parties, or pregnant people, they cannot avoid everything. Thus, strong emotions, especially anger, eventually surface.

There are many potential targets for couples' anger. For instance, if the daughter was a diethylstilbestrol (DES) baby, her mother becomes a target. Although most couples realize their doctors are not to blame for their infertility, physicians and their staff may become targets for the anger. Couples may take out their frustrations on the medical personnel because the treatment is not working. They may also be angry because the treatment is painful or because it is expensive.

Some patients will never show any negative emotion in the office. . . . After awhile I'll say to them, "You are so even-tempered. You've never said that you can't stand this anymore or anything like that." Then they tell me they're not like this at home. They cry at home. Other people will vent on the phone. Sometimes they'll yell at us because they got their period or something. Sometimes I have to get my bearings, too, and after I get off the phone I'll say to myself, "She had to vent, it's all right." You have to be in a good place as the care giver on that day. When you're getting yelled at, and even though you know it's not personal, at first you wonder why she's yelling at you. You have to really be here and listening to each patient.

Regina Matties, R.N.

During their infertility experience, couples direct their anger at many different people and things. However, they also direct most of their emotions toward themselves. They become angry that they did not start trying to conceive sooner, thinking that infertility could have been avoided. They are also angry that their bodies are failing them in this important life function.

Couples become easily angered at their loss of control over their life plan. Most couples try to plan to have their children at a certain time in their marriage. For example, many couples want children after they complete their education, their careers are on track, and the house is bought. However, infertility forces some couples to cast their plans aside.

People around us were able to plan out their lives. That I found to be real frustrating. They'd say, "I'm going to have a baby, then in two years we'll have another baby, then we'll buy a house, then we'll have a new car, and then we'll be able to build a house." They'd be able to lay out this plan and we'd think about a plan and realize we don't have that option, we haven't been able to do that.

As the infertility treatment becomes long and drawn out, couples may become angry because they have to postpone more of their education or career goals. This indefinite amount of time while waiting for something to happen can cause them to become very indecisive about future plans.

I was trying to get my master's at the same time we were trying to get pregnant. I kept delaying going on with school, because I had to make a year's commitment. And I wasn't able to do that, so I delayed finishing up. I did one year, then I delayed the second year because I kept thinking I was going to get pregnant. I delayed it for four years. It put everything in our lives on hold.

The results of the anger can be devastating. The emotion was easy to deal with when couples directed it at persons outside the family. However, more than likely, they eventually find themselves angry at each other. Communication may deteriorate and problems that once were easily solved become sources of major battles. Couples that had relationships that were happy and stable before the infertility can appear to be headed for serious difficulties.

Because of the nature of infertility and the demands placed on couples, the sexual relationship can become a battleground. Misunderstandings occur. Many fights happen around midcycle—the time when the need to succeed is greatest. The fights serve to release the stress, but also may cause the couples to avoid sex.

> Trying to conceive didn't bring us closer. There was so much stress. When I'm under stress I tend to isolate myself and just not deal with each other. I don't think it brought us closer, especially during the closest time, when you're making love and you think that it's supposed to be a very special time with closeness, and forget it. We didn't want to talk about it. We'd end up fighting when we talked about it. For a week I'd be off the wall when we'd start talking about it. Saying things like, "This is not going to work." We'd be blaming each other.

To deal with the anger, couples need to be attuned to their own and each other's feelings. They can also minimize problems if they understand that their sexual relationship and their ability to communicate will be severely stressed, despite their best intentions to stay supportive throughout the infertility. In addition, understanding the problems likely to occur and knowing that there are ways to minimize the problems, may inoculate them against some of the potential damage.

Sexual Problems

Because couples' struggle with infertility inevitably complicates their sexual relationships, working with infertile couples can be especially challenging for some counselors. Thus, it is important for counselors, clergy, and other helping professionals to be clear about their own sexual values. In addition, before working with infertile couples, counselors should understand and be comfortable with their own sexuality. Counselors should be prepared to talk openly and honestly about the ways in which infertility has created problems with couples' sexual relationships.

To increase chances for pregnancy, couples are expected to have sexual intercourse on certain days of the month and at specific intervals. Couples record the specific days that they have sexual intercourse in any given month. This allows the physician an opportunity to determine if the timing and frequency are adequate. This ritual goes on month after month without regard to either spouse's feelings, physical condition, or mood. If the day has been hard or stressful, sexual intercourse is still expected. If someone is ill, sexual intercourse is expected. If there has been an argument, both are expected to put aside their differences because intercourse remains the priority.

Many couples feel that this is a test they are in danger of failing. To compensate, couples have admitted to cheating, to having added some X's on the chart so that it would look as if their sex life is adequate. Couples may deceive the physician, but they cannot lie to themselves. They know too well which months were wasted and which months were not. As a result, romance becomes a less important aspect of the relationship. Placing the sperm into the vagina becomes the goal.

Planning becomes more complicated and thus more stressful if one partner travels some distance to work. Schedules have to be coordinated and despite, all the coordination, some couples will still miss some months. Sometimes difficult decisions are necessary.

When sex is no longer spontaneous or pleasurable, but done only with the goal of achieving pregnancy, anxiety levels rise. There is a loss of libido. Men may find it difficult to maintain an erection. Impotence is common, especially when there is a diagnosed male problem. Similarly, women may not experience orgasm.

Coping

Couples need to be able to reduce the negative impact that the sexual pressure places on their relationship. In addition, couples need to learn strategies that, first, prevent sexual problems such as temporary impotency from escalating and, second, enable them to maintain the same level of intimacy and romance they enjoyed before their infertility problems arose. There are certain things they can do to accomplish these tasks.

First, couples need to expect that there will be problems in their sexual relationship. Every act of intercourse will not end with partners telling each other that the earth moved. Women may not always have orgasms. For men, maintaining erections and completing the sex act will sometimes be difficult. If couples understand early in their infertility that their sex life will change, they may be able to reduce the resulting anxiety.

Couples also need to actively keep romance in their relationship. To accomplish this goal, they may need to change their view of romance in order to accommodate events that do not end with intercourse. Candlelight dinners, quiet nights by the fire, or walks on the beach are some examples of romantic events that need to be planned or that one partner should spontaneously suggest to the other. When these events take place, the evening does not have to end with intercourse. It certainly can, but couples have to understand that they may in fact be tired of sex. Such events communicate to each partner that they continue to care about intimacy and find each other attractive and desirable.

Couples may need to experiment with other methods of sexual intimacy. There are many methods of achieving physical pleasure in a relationship. Couples should feel free to experiment with alternative methods of stimulation such as oral or manual manipulation. Sexual positioning can change as can places where they engage in sexual intercourse. Couples might consider reading books, such as Alex Comfort's *The Joy of Sex*, that may enhance their sexual enjoyment and keep their sexual relationship exciting.

Couples can also give pleasure to each other by use of massage. There is nothing like a full body massage with a body oil to provide relaxation and to make the other feel special. Alternating turns being massaged allows each partner to experience pleasure and to have the enjoyment of giving the other pleasure.

Finally, sexual problems will arise. To effectively deal with the problems, couples will need to talk to each other about their feelings, problems, needs, and desires. The better they are able to communicate with each other, the more likely they will be able to maintain a satisfactory intimate relationship. As communication is critical in many aspects of a couple's ability to cope with infertility, the next section will discuss, in more detail, some of the basic elements of communication. If couples understand and use these ideas in their relationships, they can prevent more serious problems.

Communication Strategies

Infertility is a major stressor in couples' lives. Each partner needs to support and be supported, to handle conflicts, solve problems, and deal with the many crises that occur. The degree to which couples effectively cope with these tasks will be dependent on their ability to communicate successfully with each other during their struggle.

Effective communication is defined as the process by which a speaker sends a message to a receiver and that receiver understands the message in the way the speaker intended. Good communication results in couples' feeling understood and thus supported by each other. Good communicators are better able to solve problems and make decisions. As a result, infertile couples who value communication in their relationship will be better able to cope with the problems at each stage of their infertility. In any relationship, but especially one that involves infertility, there are many opportunities for miscommunication. When these occur, communication breaks down, problems escalate, and frustration increases. Couples can follow some guidelines that will increase their communication ability.

A Couple's Guide to Communication by Gottman, Notarius, Gonso, and Markman is an excellent resource for couples. The authors describe effective communication processes and provide ways couples can improve their abilities to express feelings, prevent conflicts from escalating, and solve problems. No doubt, if couples understand problems that are occurring, they can prevent them from developing into more difficult crises.[8]

Communication is a complex process. In any communication, there is a sender—the person who has a message to relay to another. There is also the receiver or listener—the person who is supposed to hear and interpret the message. Finally, there is the message, which involves content (what is said), affect (the emotion involved), and process (how the communication occurs). Effective communication results when the impact of the message to the receiver matches the message's intent. Thus, the speaker is understood.

Miscommunication can occur if the message sent is not clear. In such a communication, the message will frustrate, confuse, or anger the listener. Couples need to minimize the occurrence of the types of miscommunication whenever possible.

To increase the chances of being understood, speakers can communicate with "I" messages. In an "I" message, speakers take responsibility for their thoughts and feelings. For example, if the speaker has a problem with a spouse, the "I" message helps him or her communicate feelings in a way that does not cause the other to be defensive. Examples of "I" messages include

"I feel good when you listen to me."
"When you walk away from me, I feel hurt."
"I feel angry because I think I have lost control of my life."
"I am tired of going through all the tests."

Listeners have responsibility for the communication process as well. Miscommunication also occurs when the receiver does not adequately listen to the speaker. The listener may distort the message because of distraction, trying to do several things at once, or because of feelings of frustration or anger. As a result of the listener's distortions, future communication will be more difficult because the speaker is likely to become frustrated.

Active listening is a process receivers should use to communicate to the sender that they are paying attention and are attempting to understand the message. Active listening provides an opportunity to determine if the impact does indeed match the intent. If a message is not understood, active listening provides the speaker the opportunity to make the message more clear.

In active listening, the receiver relays to the sender his or her understanding of the message. The receiver does not evaluate the message or judge the speaker. The main goal in active listening is to convey to the sender that the receiver cares enough to listen to the message. More important, the receiver shows a desire to understand, to the best of one's ability, the sender's intent. Active listening can be as simple as repeating the content or the emotion from the message. It can also entail summarizing more complex messages.

Message	Active Listening
You always walk out when I am speaking. I hate that. You make me feel so bad.	You feel hurt when I walk out on you while you are speaking."
I am tired. The boss is putting pressure on me to complete my project. My secretary was complaining about all the work I was giving her. Traffic was impossible.	It sounds like you had a very difficult day. It sounds like you feel like nothing went right for you today.
You never understand. I put up with all those tests, yet you make it sound like it should be so easy for me.	It sounds like you feel that I do not understand how hard this has been on you.
I am sick and tired of you always saying we got to do what you want. You never ask me what I want to do.	You sound very angry.

To many couples, infertility seems like an endless series of frustrations, hurts, problems, and crises. Many times, one partner feels like constantly talking about problems and feelings. This can get tiring for the other partner and is not always productive. When the other begins to seem uninterested, feelings of hurt and conflict develop. As a result, anger may intensify.

To avoid such difficulties, couples can agree to structure their discussions about infertility. For example, they may want to agree to limit talks to thirty minutes each night. Specific times that meet both partners' needs could be set for the discussions. For example, couples may agree to talk for a half hour each night after dinner. There will be occasions when discussions take place at other times. However, if couples take the agreement seriously, then they can work to be effective communicators during the established time.

Couples can also limit what they talk about, especially when they are in conflict. So often discussions escalate because one or both partners bring in extraneous material that does not add anything positive to the discussion. For example, exchanging episodes of past hurts by the other will only make any conflict worse. Such a process is especially destructive when a couple is making a treatment decision. Both people have to agree early in their relationship that they will avoid such practices at all costs, even when they are most upset.

So often, couples take each other for granted. When they are involved in their own struggles, it is easy to take out their frustrations on the person about whom they care the most. So often couples can forget basic politeness, and as a result, treat their spouses in ways they would never consider treating strangers. Gottman and his colleagues discuss the importance of the social amenities in a relationship. They provide nine rules of politeness that should serve as reminders to couples:

The Don'ts of Politeness	The Do's of Politeness
1. Don't say what you can't do, or what you don't want to do.	Say what you can do and what you want to do.
2. Don't complain or nag.	Give sincere and positive appreciation. If you have an issue to resolve, set a time to resolve it.
3. Don't be selfish.	Be courteous and considerate.
4. Don't hog the conversation.	Express interest in your spouse's activities; try to listen; ask questions.
5. Don't suddenly interrupt.	Give your spouse a chance to finish speaking.
6. Don't put your spouse down.	Say things that you honestly feel and that

	you think your spouse will like.
7. Don't put yourself down.	Criticize your ideas, not yourself.
8. Don't bring up old resentments.	Focus on the present situation.
9. Don't think only of your needs and desires.	Think of your spouse's needs and desires; be empathic.[9]

Effective communication ensures that both parties treat the other with the respect deserved. Finally, each partner will feel listened to by the spouse. As a result, the relationship can be strengthened by the experience of infertility.

In contrast, ineffective communication leads to unresolved problems, escalating anger, and to people feeling hurt.

> I had an appointment with another doctor and I was going to go through with it. When I discussed it with John he said, "We really don't have the money right now." And to be honest, that really hurt me. I felt he was saying, "You don't have enough chance of getting pregnant, let's not waste the money." And it's not what he said, and it's not even what he thought, I'm sure, but that's the way I interpreted it. I thought basically, "I'm not worth it." That hurt . . .
>
> I feel that I've given up. I'm not sure that I'm going back for any treatment. I think a lot of it has to do with feeling hurt that John didn't, at that moment, want me to continue. I'm not saying he said, "Never go back." I know he doesn't want to give up on having a baby. He wants a baby, but he doesn't want to have to go through the treatment in order to get one. I don't see how he can have what he wants in both cases.
>
> I think he's afraid about my seeing a specialist for the same reason I am. I'm afraid they're going to find something that nobody else has found and say, "You can never, ever, have children no matter what you do." It would be so final. It would be difficult dealing with. It's better knowing that at least I might be able to have children.
>
> I related this whole incident to having a miscarriage. . . . At the point when he told me to cancel the appointment, something

died. I almost wished that it had been a baby because at least then I could say, "This is what died." And I don't know what died right now. But I know something is gone and I haven't been able to get it back, which is part of the reason why I haven't been able to go back for treatment. Things are different. Maybe it's the hope that died. . . . I don't think I can go on. Maybe without him pushing me to go on, it's made me feel like, "Why should I put myself through that?" If it doesn't matter that much to him, then I can't say I want to have a baby for him anymore. I don't know how much more I can go through. I do want to have the hope, but I don't know if I have it.

7

LOSS

Infertility is a continuous confrontation with loss. Initially, couples face a series of minor losses each time conception fails and menstruation begins. As the infertility persists, couples encounter more losses including the loss of control, some loss of relationships, and a loss of initial plans. Some cases of infertility involve miscarriages and stillbirths. These are more concrete losses. Finally, if the infertility reaches a time when either the physicians or the couples decide that treatment is not workable, then multiple losses, including pregnancy, a biological child, and genetic continuity must be faced. Often, these losses include a dream that was developed and nurtured from early childhood.

The feelings associated with reproductive loss, which include infertility, miscarriage, and stillbirth, can be difficult to understand intellectually. They emerge because of an emptiness or an absence of an object, rather than from the presence of something concrete. Furthermore, loss results in experiencing strong, overwhelming emotions. As a result, we never represent the full experience of loss when we attempt to describe these emotions with words. Although we attempt to use characteristics or case examples to define and describe loss, we never portray the entire meaning or emotions of the experience.

The loss of a desired object, such as a child, results in a grief reaction.[1] With grief, we mourn the loss of that loved object. In most loss experiences, including stillbirth, there is a concrete object, the baby, to mourn. In contrast, grieving over infertility and miscarriages is more complicated. In these experiences, the mourning process involves ideas, dreams, and hopes, which are abstract, and thus more difficult to understand.

Similar to infertility, grief evokes many emotions including anger, guilt, and eventually depression. As the grief intensifies, couples become more angry with themselves and others, feel more guilty, and eventually become more depressed. The cycle can seem never-ending.

Pain in grief is inevitable. One part of the grief process involves a persistent desire for the lost object. Depressive symptoms, such as sadness and a loss of pleasure, appear as the need for the object remains unfilled. The result is a sense of emptiness that can feel devastating.[2] Suicide might be contemplated as a method of making the deep hurt stop. Couples need to be reassured that no matter how bad the pain feels, it will eventually get better. They may not accept that concept immediately, but the message can eventually be heard.

Disorganization is also part of the grieving process. Couples are in a process of withdrawing emotional investment from the loved object and preparing themselves to reattach to future objects. Thus, they have fewer emotional resources left for dealing with day-to-day decisions.[3]

Withdrawal is also part of the process.[4] When grieving, individuals need time to disengage from their old patterns of interactions and to establish new ones. With miscarriage and stillbirth, couples need time to withdraw from the child they had become attached to, and ready themselves to attach to another. With infertility, couples need to withdraw from their present thoughts and fantasies of a biological child and prepare themselves for alternatives. Couples who experience loss need time to put their emotions in perspective, to reorganize and prepare to begin again.

> We had just lost our first baby. After trying to conceive for so long, we were so happy with ourselves—we finally did it. Yet, our happiness was short lived as Beth soon began to spot. When it first started, several days after Christmas, we found false reassurance from the doctor's message that bleeding was a normal occurrence and not to worry. However, when the spotting continued, our unspoken fears grew. Then, our fears became real; Beth had miscarried. When it finally happened, I suddenly found myself operating on automatic pilot. I was taking care of business, making sure Beth would be taken care of, but I never really felt it was me doing it. I felt so detached.
> As I waited for Beth to recover from her D & C, I felt so dis-

organized. Again, I was doing things, but I felt like I was some-place else. I was in more of a dream state. The feelings were not real, there was just an emptiness. I didn't know what I should do, so I just wandered around until I could see her. When she finally awoke, I felt somewhat better. I immediately did what I could to support her. At least then I was doing something real.

The hours we waited in the hospital until her discharge seemed endless. We didn't talk much—words were of no use. In the end, we were both glad to leave the hospital and go to the security of our home. When home, we spent the next couple of days in quiet, slowly trying to understand what happened and getting back the energy to begin again.

There are several reasons that grieving may be hindered in situations of reproductive loss. Infertile couples who are griev-ing the loss of their biological children are grieving for some-thing that might have been, not what was. They are grieving for the loss of a potential, not a fact. Such grief is not recognized or easily accepted by society. Couples feel hurt and frustrated that their emotions are not understood or supported by others. As a result, many couples have to resolve their loss without the sup-port that is so necessary.

The lack of certainty surrounding the reasons for the infer-tility also hinder grieving. With a large number of cases diag-nosed "normal infertility" or "diagnosis unknown", there is no known cause for the infertility. In addition, with the continuing development of new technologies and the refinement of old ones, the success rate in treating couples who are infertile is also improving. Thus, couples always have some level of hope that biological conception is possible. Friends and relatives, typically those who are uncomfortable with infertility, continually give the message that pregnancy is always possible. Thus, the grieving process is hindered by the continuing encouragement of others and maintenance of this hope.

As difficult as grief is for couples to experience, it is a neces-sary and important part of infertility. Couples experience the previous feelings of guilt and anger and have an opportunity to put them in perspective. In addition, infertile couples need to disengage from their thoughts and dreams of a biological child. They have to reattach themselves to a new sense of self and a different set of plans. They need to develop a self-esteem that is not associated with successful production of a biological child. Family continuity has to be redefined to account for several alternatives, including the possibility of no children.

Grief is also necessary on the occasion of miscarriage or still-birth. Couples, by feeling the hurt, experience the loss as real and as important. They need to take time for themselves to regroup and to reorganize their thoughts and plans. Grief time also provides couples with the opportunity to support each other and to reestablish the bonds that make relationships strong. By working through the grief together, couples can feel better about their relationship's ability to handle any difficult stress that might confront them in the future.

Miscarriage

Miscarriage, or spontaneous abortion, is a common but emotionally devastating phenomenon in medicine. After infertility, a positive pregnancy test usually brings intense joy, relief, and a sense of accomplishment. For couples, miscarriages are indeed a significant loss. For infertile couples, the loss can be especially traumatic as the couples experience a renewed and sometimes increased sense of hopelessness.

An early diagnosis of pregnancy can mean early attachment to the fetus. For some couples, bonding starts with the first missed period. They may already be thinking of names and fantasizing about the baby's appearance. In addition, they quickly tell others about their success, usually not thinking that there is a reasonable probability they may lose the pregnancy.

> I was absolutely amazed that you could develop so many feelings about it in such a short time. There was so much excitement and so much anticipation. All the thinking was into the future in those few weeks; there was really such a great attachment to that baby in that short time. Which I would never have believed if I hadn't lost it then. It was very depressing, it was very sad.

The statistics are surprising. Approximately 75 percent of all fertilized eggs never result in a live birth.[5] Of this group, 50 percent are lost before the women get their period.[6] In addition,

20 percent of women who have a recognized pregnancy indicated by a positive pregnancy test, miscarry.[7] The majority of these miscarriages occur in the first trimester.

Certain populations are at greater risk for problem pregnancies. Infertile women have a 30 percent higher risk for miscarriage, stillbirth, or intrapartum death.[8] Older women in their late thirties and early forties also are at greater risk for miscarriage.[9] Women who have had a single miscarriage are at greater risk of a second. It is true that from 20 to 30 percent of women who miscarry will most likely have more than one miscarriage. Women who have two miscarriages have a 50 percent chance of having a third.[10] After three miscarriages the probability for having another is approximately 35 percent.[11] Women who experience three or more miscarriages are diagnosed as habitual aborters. About one out of three-hundred women are habitual aborters.[12] It is encouraging, though, that approximately 70 percent who have had three or more miscarriages will eventually have a live birth. [13]

Miscarriage is often called nature's "quality control." However, research shows that 33 percent of the causes are related to maternal health. Semchyshyn believes that with the proper medical attention and care, women can prevent many miscarriages.[14]

Most physicians do not become concerned about pregnancy problems until women have experienced at least three miscarriages. Some doctors admit, and many patients agree, that physicians are slow to diagnose pregnancy problems. The physician may dismiss certain signs of miscarriage. For instance, he or she may see a small fetus on the ultrasound. Instead of believing the pregnancy is at risk, the physician will tend to believe that the woman miscalculated the date of her last period. Physicians do not always listen to or believe what their patients tell them about the early signs of miscarriage. They tend to dismiss complaints as being the worries of the overemotional.

> It was during my second pregnancy that I called my doctor about the cramps I was having. Since I had miscarried six months ago, I was very concerned. The doctor dismissed my complaint as being from eating all kinds of fruit. You know, she never even asked if I had eaten any. Because she was the doctor, I figured she knew what she was saying. I miscarried one month later.

When reasons for the miscarriage are known, they typically fall into three categories; chromosomal, hormonal, or anatomical. The cause for the miscarriage is unknown in 50 percent of cases.

Genetic problems are a significant feature in many miscarriages. They are responsible for 60 percent of miscarriages in the first six weeks of pregnancy, 15 to 20 percent in the second six weeks, and 10 percent of all miscarriages in the second trimester.[15] Most miscarriages that occur between healthy pregnancies are the result of a genetic problem.

Chromosomal abnormalities from one or both parents can place the pregnancy at risk. However, couples with normal genetic material also can have a genetic problem because of a translocation. This genetic mistake occurs when the chromosomes, which are normal, do not align in the proper order.

Physicians study couples' genetic material with a process called karyotyping. If the genetic analysis of the blood shows a chromosomal problem, then couples are usually offered the opportunity to meet with a genetic counselor. The process sounds more frightening than it is in actuality. Genetic counseling provides couples with information about the probability of having a normal pregnancy. With genetic counseling, couples are better able to make decisions regarding future attempts at pregnancy.

Hormonal problems also can cause miscarriage. As discussed earlier in the book, the uterine lining needs progesterone to nourish the developing fetus. If the lining, or endometrium, is not receiving a sufficient amount of progesterone, the fetus will not survive. Other hormonal problems that can cause miscarriage include an overfunctioning or underfunctioning thyroid gland, or a malfunctioning adrenal gland.

There are three types of anatomical anomalies that may cause miscarriage. An abnormally shaped uterus is the first type of problem. The uterus holds the fetus and provides the environment in which the pregnancy can develop. Normally, the uterus is triangular or pear-shaped. However, some women have uteri that are heart-, anvil-, or T-shaped in appearance. In any of these cases, the abnormally shaped uterus crowds the growing fetus, causing it to abort. Fortunately, the problem sometimes can be surgically repaired.

Fibroid tumors are also an anatomical cause for miscarriage.

Fibroids are benign uterine tumors consisting of muscle tissue. If the embryo begins to implant near a fibroid, it will not be able to penetrate the muscle and adequately attach itself to the wall of the uterus. A miscarriage will likely occur early in the pregnancy. Fibroids can result from adhesions left in the uterus by an intrauterine device (IUD), an abortion, or a D & C. Surgery can remove some fibroids, but inevitably, scar tissue, which also contributes to miscarriage, results from the procedure.

An incompetent cervix can also cause a miscarriage. In a normal pregnancy, the cervix holds the developing fetus in the uterus until the beginning of labor. With an incompetent cervix, the muscle at the bottom of the cervix weakens, allowing the fetus to drop out. An incompetent cervix usually occurs during the second trimester. An early sign of this problem is cramping. An internal exam will diagnose the problem. When discovered, women can have their cervix surgically sutured closed for the duration of the pregnancy.

Misshaped uteri and incompetent cervixes are the result of birth defects. Although the causes are unknown in many of these cases, the use of DES by women in the 1950s has resulted in these problems in their offspring. DES daughters are prone to T-shaped uteri. Many also are born with a shortened cervix, which places them at greater risk for problems with carrying the fetus. DES did not prove to be useful in preventing miscarriage. In fact, ironically, DES now causes the same problems in the offspring that it originally was supposed to prevent.

Certain infections also can cause miscarriage. Herpes simplex, mycoplasma organisms, chlamydia, common viruses, bacteria such as Rubella and colds, and even a high fever have been shown to result in miscarriage. These agents cause the miscarriage by infecting either the fetus or the uterine lining between the uterus and the placenta. Many infections can be successfully treated with antibiotics. However, some of these infections often show no symptoms. If the infections are not detected, they may spread to the Fallopian tubes and ovaries, causing sterility.

Recently, there has been speculation about the role of immunological causes for miscarriage. Two problems are noted in the literature. However, the area needs additional research as the data do not lead to definitive conclusions.

The first area of interest is in the blocking factor problem. Normally, the body's defense mechanism rejects foreign substances. Pregnancy, however, is the exception. The body recognizes that the embryo is different from other foreign substances, and produces antibodies that prevent the mother's white blood cells from rejecting the fetus. If the parents share certain cellular characteristics, the mother does not produce the blocking factors, and then the body attacks and eventually rejects the pregnancy.

New treatments have been developed to encourage the production of the blocking factor. A blood transfusion of leukocytes from the male is given to the female in order to help her immune system recognize fetal tissue as different and thereby not reject it. Some clinics claim a 70 to 90 percent success rate for this treatment.[16]

Autoimmune disorders also may contribute to miscarriage. An autoimmune disorder occurs when the immune system fails to recognize the embryo as its own. Antibodies attack the body's own tissue, including the nucleus of cells. With pregnancy, the site where the fetus attaches to the uterine wall can be affected, causing the body to miscarry. Although some women with an autoimmune disorder become very ill, often this disorder does not show any symptoms. As a result, the condition may be difficult to detect. When detected, however, treatment with the medication prednisone, which inhibits the activity of the body's defense system, has been used with some success.

The evidence for environmental causes for miscarriage is not consistent. There have, however, been some links between miscarriages and some of the following: toxic substances, drugs, chemicals, pesticides, computer screens, radiation, nitrous oxide, and electric blankets.[17] Research to evaluate the relationship between environmental factors and miscarriage is in process.

Some physicians believe emotions play a biological role in pregnancy. They believe that stress affects the hormone levels. Instead of prescribing bed rest, which can produce more anxiety, some doctors offer high-risk patients weekly consultations through the first trimester to help them relieve stress.

Couples experience a range of emotions immediately before, during, and after a miscarriage. A miscarriage first becomes threatened when there is an appearance of cramps and bleeding. At this point, couples usually call their physician in panic, hoping for reassurance or a miracle cure. However, doctors can do little at this point to save the pregnancy. They recommend that the woman stay calm, drink extra fluids, and rest in bed.

Couples do not find this advice soothing and become angry that the physician does not offer more medical help. In addition, they feel helpless and out of control waiting for the signs of miscarriage to stop or for their worst fears to be realized. In order to cope with their uncertainty, many couples deny their feelings and instead focus on the possible positive outcomes.

The physical signs may stop. However, problems are still possible, especially if the symptoms of pregnancy diminish. In such cases, a blood test is needed to determine if the pregnancy is viable. Furthermore, an ultrasound procedure may be used to indicate the presence of a heartbeat. If either test is negative a "blighted ovum" or empty sac may be present. Thus, pregnancy loss results.

The pain and bleeding that accompany a miscarriage can compare to those experienced in labor. Couples are easily frightened by the amount of blood and the intensity of the contractions. Women may fear life-threatening hemorrhaging or the need for a future hysterectomy. Husbands, also frightened, concern themselves with their wives' health. Together, couples fear their helplessness at not being able to control the pregnancy.

Couples usually are separated at the hospital, a time when they need each other the most. The focus is on the woman's medical needs. For the most part, little attention is given to comfort and support. Often, women are placed near the obstetrics unit. Worse, some hospitals may have women recover in the same room with others who are in the process of having their babies. This lack of sensitivity only intensifies the loss.

During the recovery period, couples feel a sense of emptiness. Women especially feel the loss as their bodies may still show signs of pregnancy. Afterward, the depression may increase as the hormones may be at the same level as those of postpartum women. But with miscarriage there is no baby. For some women, the anger and depression can be so great that they deny the miscarriage and fantasize that they are still pregnant.

I didn't think it could happen to me, so I denied it up until three or four days after I got out of the hospital. I started to deal with it later, when I had the D & C that Monday. That's probably when I really realized I had had a miscarriage. If I have a miscarriage now I know it will affect me much more, just because I'm more aware of what's going on. At the time it took a couple of days to really sink in what had happened. . . . I was still in shock, I expected everything to be just right. When you get pregnant you think the least of your worries is carrying it. Of course I'm going to carry it.

Often, doctors will sedate their patients, especially those who are crying hysterically. Physicians wrongly believe the emotional pain is too intense and that they are helping women cope with their loss. However, with sedation, they are in fact hindering the grieving process in all but the most severe cases. Pain and depression are normal and necessary as grieving runs its course.

Some couples will direct their anger at the doctor, believing that more should have been done to save the pregnancy. Intense longing for their lost babies drives chronic miscarriers to endure countless tests and treatments, insisting the doctor research every possible cause. However, many couples direct their anger toward themselves. Guilt is common. Many women question their previous behavior and wonder if they caused the miscarriage by their jogging, drinking coffee, having X rays, taking aspirin for their headaches, or having intercourse. Most doctors try to assure their patients that they cannot trigger a miscarriage. However, some continue to believe the miscarriage is punishment. The lack of medical information leads couples to blame themselves.

Sally

I'm being punished for something I did wrong. I thought I had done things right during the pregnancy, maybe it was something I neglected. Although I was reassured medically there was nothing I could have done.

Mike

Every other week there's a study coming out about something you should or shouldn't do. And one of the things is you shouldn't fly on an airplane in the early stages of pregnancy. Well, Sally had taken me away to Bermuda for my birthday. I was feeling a little guilty because she was on the plane. I don't know what studies you believe and what studies you don't. About the only thing you could do is lie down in bed and never move for nine months, as long as you don't use an electric blanket in the process.

The reactions of others to the miscarriage is usually not comforting and is often demeaning to couples. Well-intentioned friends and relatives will say things like, " You are better off, the child was probably defective," or "You'll get pregnant again." If a couple has another child, the response often is "At least you have one." Other people may feel uncomfortable talking about the miscarriage, wrongly believing that couples do not want to talk about their loss. This is usually not the case. When others ignore the miscarriage, couples feel worse. They feel that their loss has been minimized, as if it had never happened. The message many couples receive from others is that there is no cause for grief or depression. For couples, miscarriage is the death of a child. "It helps to know others view my child as real."[18]

The need for couples to grieve at this time is important. However, because there is no body or ritual for mourning this type of loss, grieving can be difficult. Many people do not realize that a baby has died. Because there is no body, for some the loss is too abstract. Even couples sense the experience as unreal, and continually question themselves about the pregnancy's existence. For infertile couples, the emotional gray area from infertility to losing a baby does not seem quite real.

There are also some long-term effects of the miscarriages that can be difficult to face. After a loss, any loss, a period of adjustment is necessary. Pregnancy loss is no different. Although couples attempt to continue with their lives as if the loss had not occurred, they will not always be successful. Anniversary dates of the miscarriage and the due dates often result in increased depression. Couples need to realize that there will be times when the feelings will reemerge. Denying the feelings' existence, no matter how painful, does not help their grieving.

We had gone to a seminar on pregnancy loss, trying to better understand the medical causes for our three miscarriages. Part of the workshop, presented by women who ran a pregnancy loss support group, discussed the emotional implications of miscarriage. As they talked about the need to mourn the loss, I began to cry, even though it was two years after my last miscarriage. In fact, I cried through the rest of the seminar, as they talked about the need for a ceremony to ritualize the loss and help make it real. I slowly realized they were talking about me and that I never adequately said good-bye to my babies.

Men have a different type of difficulty with miscarriage. They do not experience the physical symptoms of pregnancy. Often, a man does not hear the fetal heartbeat, or see his wife's extended abdomen. As a result, the pregnancy may not seem as real to him, and thus the miscarriage can be difficult to comprehend.

There is little or no social support for men at this time. Although they have also suffered a loss, men are usually left out and may even feel distant. As one man stated, "No one came to me and said, 'I am sorry.'" Because women suffer the physical effects of miscarriage, men are expected to be strong for their wives. When men do feel the intensity of the loss, they may be uncertain about if or how they can show their feelings. Men may feel that if they express their grief their wives will feel worse. However, the buried grief may surface again in the form of anger and depression.

Although we cannot discount men's reactions, women do experience the more intense feelings. Women feel as if they have let their husbands and families down. They feel embarrassed and ashamed by their failure. As with infertility, women feel inadequate that their bodies are incapable of holding a pregnancy. Miscarriages are an assault on their concept of themselves as competent women.

For some couples, the conflicting emotions can diminish their motivation for another pregnancy. They may be too afraid about the possibility of another miscarriage. Although miscarriage is a difficult event to experience, most couples are able to successfully cope with their feelings, put the miscarriage in proper perspective, and continue with their attempts to have a child.

> The miscarriages and pregnancies brought us closer together. I don't know why it did this time, there seemed to be more stress, but we seemed to pull together.

After experiencing a miscarriage couples often are hesitant to tell others right away of a subsequent pregnancy. They usually are afraid there will again be problems with their pregnancy. By not telling others, couples are limiting the amount of excitement they allow themselves to feel, thus cushioning themselves against future disappointment. In contrast, couples may be overly optimistic to guard against the anxiety that the pregnancy might again fail. For example, a couple may name their baby and set up the nursery when the woman is only four months pregnant. In any case, the early months of pregnancy are so anxiety ridden that every ache or pain signals a possible impending miscarriage. Regardless of how couples behave, pregnancy following miscarriage is less joyful.

> It's very stressful (second pregnancy). Every pain you get is worse because I get nervous. My husband wants a report at the end of the day, "What pains did you have today? Any spotting? Did you have this? Did you have that?" You just dwell on all the problems. I'm in the bathroom fifteen times a day. I can imagine all sorts of things. Last week I thought for sure I had miscarried. . . . It's very, very stressful. It's supposed to be very exciting, but it's changed. . . . I don't think I'll ever feel comfortable until the baby is born. . . . I resent it sometimes that we're constantly in this fear and can't enjoy it. . . . Especially when I look at other people's rather uneventful pregnancies, I think to myself, "Why can't I have something like that?" I resent the fact that I've been to the doctor six times already and I'm only six weeks pregnant.

Ectopic Pregnancy

An ectopic pregnancy occurs when the fetus grows outside the uterus, usually in a Fallopian tube. For that reason, an ectopic pregnancy is also called a tubal pregnancy. Many women experience the symptoms of a normal pregnancy with an ectopic pregnancy. Yet, as the embryo grows it stretches the tube, causing intense pain. It is hoped that ultrasound will diagnose the problem before it causes extensive damage to the reproductive organs. When the ectopic pregnancy is discovered, women require immediate surgery to remove the embryo. The physician may be able to save all or part of the Fallopian tube. If the tube ruptures, internal bleeding, shock, and death are possible.

Ectopic pregnancies occur in 1 to 2 percent of all pregnancies. Only 50 percent of women who have experienced an ectopic pregnancy will conceive again. Ten percent of those women will experience a second ectopic pregnancy.[19] Thus, ectopic pregnancies are emotionally draining and can have serious long-term effects.

> It's really disappointing. You get so frustrated (after five ectopic pregnancies). You ask yourself, "What do I have to do?" This is some kind of a sick joke. I can get pregnant easily, but for what? It's not where it's supposed to be and I wind up having to lose it anyway. It's hard. The fifth one was a total shock. I said, "That's it. I'm going to give up sex entirely."

Stillbirth

Still-birth is the death of the fetus in the third trimester of pregnancy or during labor and delivery. Couples usually do not think that such an event may occur. However, in 1987, there were approximately 11 infant deaths for every 1,000 live births.[20] Even though the percentage is low, the possibility of stillbirth does exist.

A stillbirth is usually caused by loss of the oxygen supply to the fetus. There are three reasons this might occur: 1) the compression of the umbilical cord; 2) the premature separation of the placenta; 3) separation of the umbilical cord from the placenta.[21] There may also be congenital abnormalities of the baby's heart or lungs, preventing the baby's breathing on its own. In roughly half of the cases of stillbirth, the cause of death cannot be determined.[22]

If the baby has died in utero, women may have to wait until labor begins, or is induced to deliver. Often, in these cases, doctors will use general anesthesia to deliver the baby, as opposed to natural childbirth. This may help reduce the emotional trauma.

Stillbirth can be one of the most heartbreaking experiences that couples face. Due to the totally unexpected nature of stillbirth, the resulting depression can be intense. The joy and excitement that the couple had experienced throughout the pregnancy suddenly turn into complete emptiness—a void. Women have an especially difficult time coping with stillbirth.

Besides feeling the failure as a result of losing the pregnancy, they also are dealing with bodily changes. Even though there is no baby, they experience the postpartum conditions of pregnancy. These hormonal changes add to the intense depression. The physical condition may delay grieving.

The grief associated with stillbirth is intense and compares to that experienced with the loss of an older child. Immediately following the stillbirth, 50 percent of couples state that they plan never to have children again. Other couples become temporarily infertile, possibly as a result of the stress and guilt. Two percent of couples choose sterilization to ensure that pregnancy does not occur again.[23] For many, this is a self imposed punishment for their failure. For others, it is an attempt to prevent themselves from experiencing such intense hurt again.

Unlike after a miscarriage, family and friends can be comforting when a stillbirth has occurred. The grieving process is more easily facilitated because there is a tangible loss over which to grieve. Couples can take some concrete actions to ease the grief. Naming and holding the child, having a memorial service with a burial are especially helpful. Although the pain is intense, these steps will help couples through the grieving process. It is hoped they will find it unnecessary to take drastic steps to prevent a recurrence of the pain.

Social Support

Despite the absence of a concrete object in many cases, reproductive loss is a devastating experience for couples. Although the intensity of different feelings may vary depending on whether the loss is from infertility, miscarriage or stillbirth, the feelings experienced will be the same regardless of the type of loss. Yet, for friends, relatives, and professionals, the pregnancy and the loss may not have seemed real. Thus, couples may not always get the recognition for their pain that they need to help them through the difficult process.

Others' lack of understanding and recognition is unfortunate for couples who experience reproductive loss. Research suggests that social support does reduce the sense of hurt couples feel after a loss. Friends who show understanding, concerned statements from physicians, and nurses who give some extra attention all make the hurt seem more bearable. For those helpers who are looking for new ways to help couples, there are no brilliant concepts. The only caveat we suggest is that helpers be able to recognize the hurt as real. A simple "I am sorry for your loss," or "If you need anything, please ask," can make a difference. In addition, many couples may need a concerned person to acknowledge and validate their pain and to be with them while they are going through the experience. Finally and most important, professionals need to be careful not to become so involved in other aspects of their professional work that they underestimate people's hurt and as a result view the extra concern and recognition for the hurt as too time-consuming and thus not necessary.

8

Resolved

When couples experience and successfully work through all the emotions of infertility, they eventually reach a time when they accept their condition. When they are at this point, they have reached the final stage of their emotional struggle—resolution.[1]

Resolution is a mixed blessing. Reaching resolution is a difficult and painful process for most couples. Furthermore, the road to resolution is filled with enormous uncertainty, bitter disagreements, and long periods of painful grief. Nevertheless, no matter how difficult the path may be, successful resolution has its own rewards. When couples reach the time when they have a mutual acceptance of their infertility, they are better able to talk about their infertility and deal with the emotions confronted. As a result, many options become open for consideration.

For successful resolution, couples need to separate their self-worth from childbearing and to separate the pregnancy experience from the desire to parent.[2] As a result of accomplishing these two tasks, they come to realize that their ideas on what constitutes a family may have changed. For some couples, remaining child-free after many years of attempting pregnancy may provide them with renewed happiness and energy. For others, conceiving a child that is partially biologically connected may be an acceptable choice. Many other couples will find happiness adopting a child that has no biological connection to them.

Couples need to understand that choosing an alternative to normal reproduction does not mean giving up or failure on their part. Counselors and other support persons need to help couples understand that there may be a time when trying to conceive is no longer hopeful or positive, but only draining and frustrating for them. Couples have to stop being "infertile" and think about getting on with their lives.

Reaching such a decision can be difficult, especially when infertile couples hear the biased comments that "having" a child is the one greatest joy in the world. However, to resolve their infertility successfully, couples need to concentrate on what is best for them and tune out these types of remarks. When successful, couples will be enlightened at their acceptance of alternatives previously rejected.

According to Menning, there are three steps or tasks that couples should engage in when coming to terms with the emotions of infertility and with achieving resolution: (1) the particular feeling is discovered and named; (2) the named feeling is honestly discussed and the origins of the feeling are discovered and worked through; (3) the person feels relief from the feeling, the feeling subsides, and the person is ready to move on to another feeling state.[3] These steps are necessary at each stage of the infertility experience. The faster couples can engage in these steps, the sooner they will be able to accept their condition.

Reaching resolution is a slow process because accomplishing the tasks described by Menning can be arduous. At each stage, couples may have one or more issues that are specific to themselves and their situation. The length of time necessary to deal with the issues will depend on their importance to the couple. Thus, these issues become blocks to resolution and prevent the couple from moving on. A block may occur in any of the stages of infertility and may last for varying degrees of time. However, as couples are able to face and overcome each block, they move that much closer to accepting their infertility.

Although the blocks may differ from couple to couple, there are some common ones which are typically encountered. Issues during the denial stage can be most difficult to overcome. For most, denial is a short-term process. However, if couples find themselves refusing a diagnosis and thus putting off the initial treatments for an extended period of time, they may have more serious problems to overcome. For the most part, couples stuck in denial have their self-esteem so connected with producing a child that it is too traumatic to accept infertility. As a result, they continually look for physicians who will tell them that nothing is wrong.

Blocks in anger are more common. For the most part, we are reared to control our anger, and thus do not know how to respond well to the emotion when it emerges. With infertility and all the unfairness associated with it, anger is unavoidable. However, if individuals have never been taught to express their anger, they may need assurance that their feelings are appropriate and a necessary part of successfully dealing with their condition.

Anger can be especially frightening for some couples. They may be afraid that the marriage could not withstand the feelings they are experiencing if expressed. Such couples typically are not accustomed to arguing or giving negative feedback to each other. As a result, both partners keep their feelings to themselves. Thus, they never have the opportunity to work through this stage.

Denial and anger are just two examples of blocks that can occur. Couples who understand that blocks can occur will be better able to recognize them when they are encountered. Furthermore, they will be ready to overcome them and thus successfully deal with the emotions as they surface.

When couples successfully resolve their infertility, they are able to handle the emotions and integrate them into their entire infertility experience. When they achieve this stage, the feelings will not disappear, but instead, are more easily confronted when they again emerge.

Couples, as a result of resolving their infertility, are able to reevaluate their life goals and thus choose an alternative to conception that best helps them reach those goals. With resolution, couples can achieve the contentment and peace of mind that had alluded them during their previously infertile years. They are able to see that the alternatives previously dismissed as unacceptable can in fact bring happiness.

> Four years ago, I decided I could never adopt a child. To me, adoption meant admitting failure and allowing my infertility to get the best of me. At the time, I was too caught up in the battle and less concerned about having a child. Of course I didn't realize that then.

Eventually, my values and outlook changed. I slowly began to understand that parenting was most important and that conception was only one way toward that means. I was then able to see more clearly the happiness others were having with their adopted children—it did not differ from the experiences of my fertile friends. Wait, it was different—better in some cases.

At some point, and I don't know when, I started focusing on adoption. Although we were continuing treatment for our infertility, the success of the treatments became less important. Our lives no longer revolved around whether or not I was getting my period. At this point, I felt I finally accepted our infertility and was ready to get down to the business of becoming a parent through some other means.

Pregnancy

The most wanted culmination to infertility is, of course, pregnancy. Couples anticipate hearing those wonderful words, "You are going to have a baby." However, some may not realize that pregnancy after an infertility struggle does not always mean bliss.

Couples assume that the achievement of pregnancy will solve all their emotional problems associated with infertility. Some may expect pregnancy to take away the anger, grief, and guilt that they experienced during their infertile years. Some may also be disappointed that pregnancy did not bring all the satisfaction that they desired. Although this long-awaited event will bring the child that couples hoped for, with the pregnancy come new anxieties and concerns.

For many couples, news of a positive pregnancy test does not mean happiness and excitement alone. For some, their first feelings may be denial. Because they are fearful of another disappointment, similar to those they experienced month after month during their infertility, they may deny that pregnancy has happened. At the extreme, some couples have conditioned themselves to be so pessimistic about the occurrence of pregnancy that they never believe, or get excited, until after the baby arrives. As a result, they will not seek medical care for months. More typically, couples may not prepare for the baby in the usual manner by purchasing baby clothes and furniture for the nursery. Women may put off buying maternity clothes until the very end of their pregnancy, when they have no choice—all to protect against the hurt that has accompanied so many of their attempts to have a child. As an example, when one woman was asked when her baby was due she was very surprised by the question. She wondered how that person knew she was pregnant. She surely did not believe it showed because she herself could hardly believe she was pregnant.

Many couples find it hard to accept attention and congratulations when others learn that they are expecting a child. This new-found attention usually comes from family and friends who may not have been as supportive or sensitive about the couple's infertility problems. The attention may stem from the fact that more people have been through parenting and can now offer un-solicited advice based on their parenting experiences. In general, people are more comfortable discussing pregnancy and children than infertility.

The isolation from the fertile world that was previously experienced is not immediately overcome when infertile couples achieve pregnancy. Even though they are not technically infertile anymore, couples who have been outside the fertile group for so long do not feel an automatic association with other fertiles. Even by attending exercise class for pregnant women and other meetings for pregnant women, some women still find it difficult to identify with other mothers. Some will still consider themselves infertile.

Some couples will terminate contact with their infertile friends out of fear of provoking jealousy. Others may not want to be around their infertile friends so they can repress some of those old feelings associated with their infertility. Thus, they believe they will be able to enjoy the pregnancy. However, losing old friends can be upsetting and makes the pregnancy less enjoyable.

Infertile women react differently to their pregnancy. Physically, being pregnant may not be exactly as the woman had fantasized during her struggle with infertility. Those who expected to be constantly "glowing" may complain angrily about normal discomforts, thinking that their previous infertility exempts them from nausea, backaches, and water retention. In contrast, some women forbid themselves the luxury of complaining at all. They feel very guilty if they even think about complaining and therefore do not express their natural feelings. Some may carry this through to parenting and feel that they cannot get angry at their child. These women feel that by expressing negative feelings, either during the pregnancy or to the child, makes them appear ungrateful.

A pregnancy for infertile couples will not end old marital difficulties and will often present new problems to the marriage. Studies show that there is an increased risk of psychological problems, including self-image problems, anxiety, and unrealistic expectations about pregnancy and parenthood, if there are unresolved marital issues still present at the onset of pregnancy.[4] Infertile couples emotionally drained by their experience may believe they can be less supportive now that the struggle has ended. On the contrary, the worry of losing the pregnancy, and the strain it puts on each of the partners, can cause considerable tension and anxiety. As a result, infertile couples will need to continue the emotional support for each other throughout pregnancy.

Couples' sexual relationship may still suffer during pregnancy as it did during infertility. During infertility, sex became a timed event. Now that pregnancy has been achieved, couples may think that everything will be back to normal. However, many couples may be tired of sex, finding it no longer brings the excitement of their preinfertility days. Couples will need time to redevelop some of their old desires and sexual practices. Furthermore, pregnancy introduces some new obstacles into the sexual relationship. The hormonal changes that occur can sometimes lower a woman's sex drive. She may also feel that she is not particularly attractive in her present condition so she may not feel very sexual. There may also be a very real fear, for both partners, that they may harm the baby during intercourse.

Pregnancy may actually cause old feelings of inadequacy and failure to resurface. Problems during pregnancy, labor, or delivery may bring back old infertile feelings of being defective and out of control. If the pregnancy was achieved through artificial insemination by a donor (AID) or a surrogate situation, one or both of the partners are still infertile. They must learn to deal with their feelings regarding the baby's conception.

Another problem that may arise is when it becomes time to

think about having a second child. Couples are now faced with other questions regarding their previous infertility. How easy or difficult will it be to conceive a second child? Will it happen at all? Some couples must deal with the issue of either trying to conceive spontaneously or assuming they are still infertile.

Pregnancy after infertility can present new problems and does not always take care of the old ones. For couples who thought they would be living in a fantasy world, or that all their problems would be solved by the pregnancy, the reality of paying bills and mowing the lawn still exists. Even though the stress of infertility ends with the arrival of the child, the pressures of everyday life go on.

Adoption

Adoption is a commonly used alternative to having a biological child. Twenty-five percent of infertile couples are choosing adoption as an option to their infertility.[5] The National Committee for Adoption estimates that more than 60,000 adoptions by nonrelatives had taken place in 1986.[6] Approximately 2 to 4 percent of the North American population is adopted.[7] For many couples adoption can be a wonderful alternative in building a family.

Nevertheless, adoption should be a choice freely made by couples and not something assumed to be the next logical thing to do when infertile. For instance, some couples may interpret adoption as defeat in their battle with infertility. These couples believe that adoption is a symbol to society of their inadequacy in reproduction and an announcement of failure. By agreeing to adoption, couples wrongly believe they are giving up on their quest for pregnancy. In addition, they think that adoptive parenthood will be viewed as different from biological parenthood, and the child viewed as "second best." Well-meaning friends and relatives may offer adoption as a consolation to infertility: "Never mind, you can always adopt." Other comments such as "I could never love someone else's child" may leave the couple feeling confused about their decision. However, couples can turn adoption into a special opportunity to parent a child that is not biologically related to them, but is, in fact, their child.

> We wanted to be parents and complete our family. It didn't
> matter how we got there. Neither of us felt hooked to our genes.
> It (adoption) seemed right for us.

Infertile couples report three general themes that upset them
when they consider adoption. First, many believe that others
think the bonding and love that occur in adoption are second-
rate. For some, the biological tie is important for bonding and
love. Comments from others about not understanding how couples could love a child that was not their own only serve to
reinforce this thinking. Adoptive mothers have reported that
biological mothers denigrated their feelings and experiences as
mothers.[8] These biological parents perceived their love for their
children as more intense and therefore better. Thus, despite the
large number of adoptions, society continues to label it as different, and thus not so good as biological parenting. As a result,
infertile couples believe parenting an adopted child will be considerably more difficult and less rewarding than it would be with
a biological child.

Secondly, many infertiles believe that others view the adopted
child as second rate because of the unknown genetic past. For
some, the child is considered inferior because of a "suspect"
genetic background. Many of these couples falsely believe they
are going to create the perfect child through a pregnancy. However, more than likely, they have failed to research their own
gene pool. Furthermore, negative responses from couples' families about the disruption of their own biological lineage and the
so-called "bad blood theory" put additional pressure on couples
who consider adoption.[9] An adopted child in this type of family
would have difficulty measuring up to the adoptive parents'
expectations.

Finally, the most prevalent misconception about adoption is
that the adoptive parents are not the real parents. Some infertile
couples believe that the nine months of pregnancy are more
important than the eighteen years of rearing a child. The message that infertile couples feel they frequently receive from the
fertile world is that a biological tie is a prerequisite for parenthood or a loving relationship.[10] Comments such as "After you
adopt, you will probably have children of your own" or when a
biological child is described as their "own" exemplify this be-

lief.[11] However, the majority of adoptive parents feel that adoption satisfies their desire to have a child, and they consider the child as their own.

> We consider it our obligation to teach them. We understand that most people aren't as far along as we are on this (adoption). They haven't experienced the pain we went through when we couldn't have a child.

Some couples may not be able to separate the act of reproduction from that of parenting. The presence of an adopted child, instead of being a joy, may be a constant reminder of their infertility. For couples who have not mourned the loss of a biological child, adoption will not be a satisfying substitute. Even though they go through the adoption process, they lack a sense of entitlement to their adopted child.[12] As a result of their poor psychological adjustment to their infertility, these couples may have difficulty disclosing the adoption to others and to the child.[13] These couples would also be in danger of having problems parenting their adopted child.

Many adoptive parents put themselves through considerable personal torment after they adopt. Many try, through adoption, to regain the loss of control they have felt during their infertility. When pregnancy has failed, they try to prove their success in parenting. They place more stress on themselves by trying to be "perfect parents." They will not complain about the typical problems parents face such as sleepless nights. Furthermore, when the child is not "perfect" and displays behavior such as tantrums, they feel inadequate. Their sense of failure is quickly rekindled.

Adopted children are in danger of developing specific problems.[14] Some children may go through a period of confusion about their identity and may feel rejected by their birth parents. At the same time the adoptive parents fear that the child will eventually want to meet his birth parents and they will lose the child's love in the process. However, for children, the genuine feelings of parental love, or lack of it, will eventually have more impact on their development than will their awareness of being adopted.

> Tommy will never know a time when he didn't know he was adopted. I want it to be a natural part of his upbringing: His

name is Tommy; he lives in Florida; he's adopted; he goes to
school . . . we don't want to negate the difference between adoptive birth and natural birth. The crucial thing is we're a family.

Adoption can cause many different reactions from the adoptive parents as well as from others. Feelings of mutual jealousies
may arise. Friends may mistakenly envy adoption as the easy way
out from the pains of labor. Adoptive parents envy the way
fertile friends may control the spacing of their children, as they
cannot. In addition, there are only a handful of enlightened
companies that have leave benefits and subsidies for adoption.
All these issues should be resolved at the time the adoption plan
is developed.

The well-known myth about a guaranteed pregnancy after
you adopt is just that—a myth. Statistics show that only about 5
percent of infertile couples become pregnant after they adopt,
and they would have conceived anyway.[15] There may always be a
sadness about not experiencing pregnancy. Those feelings can
be expected even from the best-adjusted adoptive parents.
Those feelings should not be denied, just put into proper perspective.

Adoption is an opportunity to turn the negative experience of
infertility into a positive one. The many couples who have
adopted children quickly realize that they would not have their
child if not for their infertility. The anger, sadness, and guilt
become gratitude toward their infertility. The happiness in their
lives makes the past feelings from their struggle with infertility a
blur.

The final weeks waiting for our child was as bad as anything we
went through. I was worthless at work, knowing that the call could
come at any time. A friend, understanding my anxiety because he
had adopted two children, told me that once I got the child, the
worry would quickly be forgotten. When he said it, I didn't really
believe him.

We eventually got the call and made the necessary arrangements to get our child. The moment I took my son into my arms,
the pain and anxiety disappeared. For the first time in eight years,
my life was completely filled with bliss. There was nothing better.
All the years of infertility were no longer relevant. If I had an
opportunity to trade the pain of the eight years for our child, I
wouldn't do it. Our child was worth the wait.

The Adoption Process

Agency Adoption

Although there are several different methods couples may use to adopt a child, the most popular is the traditional agency adoption. In this approach, couples apply for adoption with an established agency. There are many public and private agencies providing adoption services in the United States. Reputable agencies are licensed and state regulated. Agencies charge a fee usually based on a percentage of the couple's annual income. The average fee is $10,000.

Agencies typically have requirements that adoptive couples must meet in order to be considered as prospective adoptive parents. For example, one of the major restrictions is age, with many agencies maintaining an upper level of 40 years for the older partner of the adopting couple. One couple had been turned down not only because of her age, but also because of the husband's weight. In addition, most agencies require that a home study be undertaken by a certified social worker. A home study is a description of the couple's home with a detailed psychosocial history of both partners. The home study typically requires couples to answer many personal questions about their income, feelings toward their infertility, motivations for adoption, and their marital relationship. Many couples feel threatened by the home study and angry that couples who conceive are not subject to the same requirements. Couples again experience a loss of control while they are waiting to be judged suitable or unsuitable to parent. Many couples find that they have to pass a series of tests in order to be accepted for this type of adoption.

Many couples, providing they are accepted, like the contentment that comes from knowing that the agency is doing all the work and they can take a break for awhile. Agency adoptions also, to a large degree, offer couples a certain amount of emotional protection. They safeguard couples against the possibility of a failed adoption by making sure all the legalities are handled before couples receive their babies.

Another major drawback to agency adoptions, besides the stringent requirements, is the long wait for a healthy newborn. An increase in the number of abortions along with more social acceptance for teens or unwed women who keep their babies has reduced the number of infants available to agencies. The average wait is from three to seven years.

If a couple is willing to take a child who belongs to a minority group, toddler, or a physically or emotionally handicapped child, the placement can be made almost immediately. These adoptions cost far less, and medical and counseling expenses are usually subsidized.

Foreign Adoption

With the wait for newborns at some agencies being as long as seven years, many couples have found traditional adoptions too frustrating to consider. In addition, because other couples do not meet some of the requirements related to age, weight, or marital status, agency adoptions are not a viable option. As a result, international adoptions have become popular, especially for those who are not comfortable with the work or risk involved with independent adoptions.

In 1986, The National Committee for Adoption estimated that 15 percent of the adoptions were of foreign-born infants.[16] South Korea, Chile, Peru, and Columbia are just some of the countries that provide babies for the United States. In many cases, countries have an overabundance of children who would be destined to reside in orphanages. Thus, these countries make contracts with agencies in the United States to broker the adoptions. International adoptions are an example of how everyone can benefit from a solution.

In many cases, foreign adoptions are similar to traditional agency adoptions. A home study is usually required. In some cases, a psychological evaluation may also be needed. The difference, and thus the advantage, of international adoptions is the short waiting list. Couples can receive a baby aged four weeks to six months from a foreign adoption service in six months or less. The fee averages around $12,000.

Foreign adoptions are not without their problems. In many cases, the circumstances of the birth are unknown. The medical history of either birth parent may be unavailable. In addition, the pre- and postnatal care may have been inadequate or nonexistent. Problems at birth occur more frequently. Health problems can be expected and couples should be ready to cope with them if they do occur.

International adoption is not for couples who need to have a child with their physical characteristics because there is a greater likelihood of significant differences. In such cases, the children and the couple would always be reminded of the adoption or infertility issues. These adoptions can be very successful and rewarding, but couples would need to have resolved their infertility and also be ready to openly deal with the children concerning their adoption.

In many cases, especially with South American adoptions, couples must travel to the country of the child's birth to receive the baby. It is common for couples to wait for many weeks while the legal system of the country completes its task of formalizing the surrender and allowing the child to leave the country. There are cases where couples saw their babies, left the country, and then waited another six months or more to receive their infants. American couples may not be ready for the pace and the laws that move the systems in these countries. There are also cultural differences that make the process more frustrating. Finally, as the couples are in a foreign country, they are more prone to be taken advantage of by people who understand how important the adoption is for the couple. Foreign adoption can be very satisfying, but couples must go into the process with an understanding of the problems that may be encountered.

Independent Adoption

Birth mothers and infertile couples have been increasingly disenchanted with the traditional agency approach to adoption. Birth parents want more control over whom they choose to parent their child. Couples looking to adopt are becoming very frustrated with the rules and requirements imposed by agencies. As a result, birth mothers and infertile couples alike are being drawn in greater numbers to independent or private adoption.

Couples begin the private adoption process by locating a birth mother. They may do this either by word of mouth or by sending letters to obstetricians, abortion counselors, or college campuses. Placing ads like the following in the personal section of various newspapers is becoming common.

Loving, secure couple wishes to provide a home for a precious infant. We yearn for the day when we hear the patter of little feet in the nursery. Let us help each other. Medical and Legal fees paid. Call Collect.

Attorneys are another source for infants. There are lawyers who have developed a reputation for being involved with adoptions and thus have access to birth mothers. Although there are many reputable attorneys who provide adoptions services, couples must understand that a black market does exist in the field. If a professional states that a couple can get an infant in a short period, but for a substantial fee, they should be wary, despite the attraction of such an offer. Couples should seek out attorneys who are knowledgeable about private adoption and have sound reputations.

There are also consultation services available for both birth mothers and prospective adoptive parents. For a fee, they guide couples in the process of locating and making contact with birth mothers. They may also place the advertisements for the couples in areas known to have high rates of single parent births. At the same time, they may help birth mothers find shelter for the duration of their pregnancies and help them to decide on suitable couples to adopt their children. If couples do not want to be called at home, this service may act as a phone contact for them.

Laws vary across states in regard to private adoptions. Some states are highly restrictive, while others are only concerned about regulating fees. Most states allow medical and legal costs to be paid to the birth mother by the adoptive parents. Some areas also allow for parents to pay reasonable living expenses to the birth mother.

In contrast to public perception, the expenses involved with private adoption can be less than if the couple made use of an agency. Some birth mothers may have medical insurance to cover prenatal care and the delivery fees. Sometimes the adoptive parents' insurance will cover the baby's hospitalization. If the birth mother changes her mind, however, there is a risk of losing money that was to be paid before delivery. Many couples believe the risk is worth taking in order to get a child quickly.

After a couple makes contact with a birth mother, usually by phone, a brief résumé about the prospective adoptive parents' life-style, along with a picture, is sent to the birth mother. If the birth mother believes the couple is appropriate for her child, a meeting may be arranged. Some birth mothers and/or couples do not want to meet, but do continue to communicate either by phone or through an intermediary. Some may want to leave everything for their attorneys to handle. Whatever all parties are comfortable with is acceptable. Couples have to decide early in the process how involved they will be with the birth mother. Sometimes their feelings will change.

> Mr. and Mrs. Peters began the adoption process with the belief they would have limited involvement with the birth mother. When they received the call, and concluded the introductions, they reluctantly agreed to meet with her. After that initial meeting, they found themselves becoming more and more attached. The phone calls increased. They visited her several times, staying at her apartment. By the end of the pregnancy, they became a source of support for the woman and contact was daily. They became the birth mother's labor coach, were in the delivery room when their child was born, and spent every day with the birth mother and the baby while both were in the hospital. For them, the birth and subsequent adoption became more special than they had ever imagined possible.

Depending on the specific arrangements made, the prospective adoptive parents will be notified either when the birth mother goes into labor or after the baby is born. Usually they are allowed to take the baby home from the hospital or shortly thereafter.

The legal adoption process is a two part procedure. First, the biological parents terminate their rights to the child. The length of time that they have to surrender the child varies from state to state. In some states they may surrender the child immediately. In others, the process can take up to two weeks. It is preferred if the birth father signs the termination consent, but in many cases, he is either unknown or unavailable. In such cases, additional steps may be required prior to finalization of the adoption.

The second step in the process is the finalization of the adoption. This occurs in the adopting parents' county and usually takes place not less than six months after the surrender. At finalization, a judge validates the adoption decree and reissues a birth certificate in the adoptive parents' family name. This adoption decree is the same regardless of whether the process occurred privately or through an agency.

One of the major advantages of independent over agency adoptions is the length of the waiting period. The average time for a couple to bring home an infant after initiating an independent process is one year. Some independent adoptions have been known to occur in as little time as three weeks.

Another positive aspect of independent adoption is the possibility of contact with the birth mother. Even if contact is through an intermediary, couples have unique access to the birth mother that is usually not available in agency adoptions. Thus, they have access to considerable amounts of personal and medical data. Couples can ask questions and are able to get important information about their child's biological history. Such information can be very useful when the child is older.

In some cases, the couple and birth mother develop a special relationship that benefits all parties through the pregnancy. For the couple, they are able to evaluate the birth mother's feelings prior to the surrender and may be able to anticipate the possibility that the adoption may not succeed. They are able to experience the pregnancy through the birth mother, an experience denied them because of their infertility.

For the birth mother, she gets additional support from the couple. Furthermore, she gets a sense of the family to whom she is giving her child. She also sees the happiness she is giving to others and experiences firsthand the appreciation the adopting couple has for her. This joy makes her own feelings of loss easier to manage.

There are also some risks that go with independent adoption. Most importantly, the birth mother may change her mind. Any agreements made during the pregnancy prior to the legal surrender are not binding. Couples can lose any monies paid. In addition, couples need to understand the emotional devastation that may result. Couples begin to attach to the hoped for child early in their relationship with the birth mother. A failed adoption, especially if there was extended contact, would create as severe a loss as any miscarriage or stillbirth experience.

Couples also must be prepared for a child with health problems. Just as the birth mother is not bound to an agreement, neither are the prospective adoptive parents. If a child is born with a medical problem, the adopting parents need to decide if they will accept that child. Given the hopes that have developed for the child, the money already paid, and their dreams for a perfect child, the decision is not clear-cut.

Couples who advertise face the additional risk of being victimized. Because infertile couples have suffered for so long, they tend to be driven in their attempts at adoption. As a result, they are vulnerable to exploitation, greed, and manipulation. The black market is one way people take advantage of a couple's desire for a child. However, there are more subtle ways as well. There are stories of birth mothers working with several couples at once, only to make her final decision at the last moment based on her best offer. Other times, people exploit the couple's desperation by offering something—a baby that doesn't exist—in hopes of getting money.

Private adoption seems fairly easy and straightforward. However, because of the risks, it is not for couples who cannot handle the involvement and uncertainty that are part of the process. Many couples eventually go back to agency or international adoption after one or more failed attempts with the private process. Success in private adoption is only measured one way, by bringing home a child. Although problems may have occurred along the way, they are quickly forgotten once the final adoption decree is signed.

> After watching our friends successfully adopt privately, we decided to begin the process. We prepared our résumé, advertised in recommended papers, spread the word through other sources, and then waited. After three months, we finally got our first call. It was at 11:30 pm. We were ecstatic. After sending our résumé to the birth mother, we made a second, then a third, contact. The relationship was developing beautifully. She even wrote and sent us a picture of herself and the birth father. We sent her flowers for Valentine's day and some money for expenses—she was very poor. She thanked us for the money (she never asked for it) and never made a big deal about it. Our relationship developed over the next six weeks through frequent

phones calls. We all agreed that we should meet, so we prepared to visit her, bought plane tickets, made hotel reservations, all with her consent and enthusiasm.

As the date for our meeting drew near, the situation became very bizarre. She gave us several excuses as to why we could not meet, including threats to her life by the birth father. The details are too unbelievable to discuss here and are probably worthy of a short story. Through a series of calls we made, we discovered the girl was not pregnant and was using us for reasons we still do not fully comprehend. Needless to say, we were crushed.

We recovered and continued our search for a child. We talked about the steps we would take in the future, to avoid another devastating experience. We continued with the process, more cautiously and certainly more wisely.

We received a second lead, this time through a friend. We established contact with the birth mother through a third party. We had mixed feelings because, despite the problems of the last attempt, we liked the relationship that could potentially develop with more direct contact. We believed that meeting the birth mother would be a positive benefit for our potential child. However, we accepted the relationship because we knew we would accept anything that might bring us our longed-for child.

After three months of anxiety and uncertainty, we got THE CALL—our child was born. We traveled the next day and after thirteen hours of driving, we held our son for the first time. Luck was on our side this time, as the hospital allowed us to room in with our child from the moment we arrived. There are no words to describe the joy we experienced during those next sixty hours while we cared for our son in the hospital. However, it gets even better. Although we never expected to meet the birth mother, she decided she wanted to give our son a present. She came to our room unexpectedly on our last day in the hospital. The next five minutes were tense, everyone was crying, but the result was a picture of our son, his adoptive mother, and his biological mother. This is a memory worth all the pain experienced through the infertility and the previous failed adoption. We got our dream—and more.

Artificial Insemination by Donor

Artificial insemination by donor (AID) is a legitimate option for couples when the male has an untreatable problem and the female is considered fertile. Approximately 5 percent of couples attempt AID each year, which results in between 15,000 and 20,000 births.[17] For many couples, AID provides the answer to their dreams of having a child.

AID is a straightforward procedure whereby sperm, anonymously donated, is injected into the uterus during the women's fertile period. Women are asked to monitor their basal body temperature for several months prior to the procedure in order to determine ovulation. Sixty percent of couples achieve pregnancy within six months.[18]

The donor is usually selected in order to match the race, blood type, and eye and hair color with the husband. Clinics will vary in the degree to which they screen donor sperm for sexually transmitted diseases, hepatitis B, and genetic abnormalities. Thus, it is important that couples become involved with only reputable programs.

Although the procedure is relatively simple, it is not without psychological complications. One woman described AID as rapelike.[19] When comparisons are made, the two have some similarities. For instance, in both cases, women lack control over their bodies, while a stranger's semen is inserted into the uterus.

Despite its growing popularity and acceptance as a method of having a child, the decision to utilize the procedure can be difficult. Couples need to consider many issues.

First, legal issues need to be researched and resolved. Many states do not have laws governing AID, and as a result legal questions in regard to the offspring are unclear. Some states consider AID as adultery. Thus, couples considering AID should be advised to consult an attorney as part of their decision-making process.

Religious issues may also be a consideration for some couples. While most religions have taken a neutral position in regard to AID, the procedure is forbidden by the Roman Catholic Church and in Orthodox Judaism. For those couples whose religious beliefs are important, consulting a trusted clergy is recommended. For those clergy that work with couples who ask about AID, it is important to understand the couples' dilemma. Clergy can discuss their religion's position on AID while at the same time being nonjudgmental and providing the necessary support to couples.

Finally, emotional factors need to be successfully resolved. Couples should work through issues regarding their infertility. Resolving their infertility is particularly important for men, as they have the most reluctance about the procedure. Clinical experience indicates that women seem to be more certain about their desire to attempt AID.[20] In contrast, AID confirms the loss of genetic continuity for many men. Furthermore, men tend to feel more isolated and left out by the AID procedure.[21]

However, the AID procedure is not viewed negatively by all men. Many have a sense of relief that they have this option. For them AID is a way around a problem. They are glad that something can be done and are happy that at least 50 percent of the child's genes are from the couple.

Indeed, couples should be assisted in understanding the positive aspects of AID. They should include the following advantages along with the problems in their discussions when considering AID.

1. the woman will experience pregnancy and birth,
2. the couple can ensure the prenatal care of the baby,
3. the infant will have 50% of the couple's genetic makeup,
4. the couple can have a child without the problems and costs associated with adoptions.[22]

It is common, too, for couples to delay making the decision to enter an AID program. Given the complexity of the issues involved, it is understandable that couples do not rush into AID. In fact, many AID programs prescreen clients to determine their psychological readiness for the procedure. As with any difficult decision, couples should be advised to consider all the issues and come to a mutual resolution that is agreeable to both individuals. As couples place considerable hope in the success of the procedure, stress and anxiety are expected for days prior to the insemination. Open communication during this time becomes important. In addition. it is helpful to both partners when husbands are present for the inseminations. Not only does their presence provide support, but men feel that by accompanying their wives for the inseminations, they are participating in the procedure.

AID is a highly emotional experience, even after pregnancy

has been achieved. There is a constant worry during the pregnancy, especially for women. They worry about the donor—wondering if a mistake was made in screening the donor, especially with regard to physical characteristics. They also worry about the health and intelligence of the child.

Men typically have different feelings regarding a pregnancy achieved through AID. Some husbands are jealous of the donor because it was his sperm and not the husband's that was able to help his wife conceive. There may be a sense of competition with the donor which then results in some latent, unconscious anger. It is for these reasons that it is critical that the couple work out these feelings prior to undergoing the procedure. On a more positive side, experience indicates that most men do successfully deal with their feelings. They are usually very supportive of their wives throughout the pregnancy, attending childbirth classes and participating during the delivery.

Even after the difficult decision of choosing AID as an option, further issues need to be considered. Most couples, on the recommendation of their physician, choose not to tell anyone about conceiving by AID. It is believed that secrecy protects the couples from others' insensitivity. However, by choosing not to tell others, they also isolate themselves from some important support systems.

Finally, and very importantly, couples need to determine whether they will tell their children about how they were conceived. In the past, the common practice was to keep AID secret. However, there is a trend toward openness, although not to the degree that occurs with adopted children. It is not clear how children adjust psychologically after being told they were conceived through AID. However, if children discover the truth by means other than from their parents, it can be predicted that problems will occur. Like the other issues regarding AID, there are no clear answers.

Surrogate Birth Mother

A more controversial solution that is chosen by some couples is surrogate motherhood. Surrogacy is somewhat similar to AID in that a third party is used to conceive a baby. Artificial insemination is performed on the surrogate, using the husband's sperm. When conception occurs, the surrogate carries the child to term and then, as with adoption, surrenders the parental rights after the birth. Surrogate arrangements have been highly sensationalized in the media and are complicated by many ethical, emotional, and legal issues.

Although some couples search for a surrogate by newspaper advertisement, many work with agencies that deal specifically with surrogacy. Some of these surrogate agencies provide everything for couples, including matching the surrogate to the couple, and legal and psychological counseling for both the couples and the surrogate. These programs will also perform the inseminations, provide prenatal and postpartum care, and make the delivery arrangements. The costs involved can be as high as $50,000. Surrogate mothers usually receive $10,000 for their participation.

After choosing surrogacy, couples need to decide their level of involvement with the surrogate mother. Couples can either choose to meet the surrogate or may want to remain anonymous. Couples can select the surrogate themselves or leave that decision to the attorney or agency.

If couples choose to meet the surrogate mother, they may develop a positive emotional bond. Through this bond, couples may be allowed to follow the pregnancy rather closely. They may even become the surrogate's birthing coaches and be present for the delivery. The infertile women may look forward to buying maternity clothes for the surrogates and watching the pregnancies progress. Some wives enjoy this close relationship. They are able to experience the pregnancy vicariously through the surrogate.

With surrogacy, as with AID, the baby has 50 percent of the couple's genetic makeup. In some rare cases, the wife's egg may be fertilized through IVF but is transferred to the surrogate. Thus, the child has all the genes from the couple. However, there are also some negative aspects to surrogacy. Most important, the surrogate may decide to keep the child. However, the husband, because he is the biological father, could petition the court for custody. The financial and emotional expense of such a fight could be more than couples had planned.

There are very few laws governing surrogate arrangements. Contracts are signed but they are usually based on trust and not enforceable in a court of law. Rarely is the surrogate mother ordered by the court to surrender the child. As a result, couples involved with surrogates are very vulnerable to last-minute changes by the biological mother. If the surrogate reluctantly surrenders the baby she may place some demands on the couple, such as continued contact with the child and visitation rights. Because all parties were less emotionally involved before the pregnancy and birth, the couple may not have considered these demands when developing the original contract.

If the surrogate miscarries or has a stillbirth, the couple will experience the emotional loss typically associated with any pregnancy. However, they also lose the sizable downpayment given to the surrogate when the agreement was instituted.

Surrogacy may be emotionally difficult for infertile women. For instance, the couples' sex lives are again invaded. In order for the inseminations to be successful, husbands may have to abstain from intercourse with their wives during certain times. As a result, wives may become angry that their sexual schedules are being disrupted by this outside party. In addition, they can become jealous of the surrogates' ability to conceive their husbands' babies. Their feelings of inadequacy may resurface again.

A couple should be aware of the surrogate's understanding of surrogacy and the motivations for agreeing to the process. Some surrogates do not know what they are getting involved with when making the decision. The emotional attachment to the baby can become very strong, and thus the desire to keep the child will also be strong. In addition, the surrogate mother is usually criticized by family and friends for her voluntary decision to conceive a baby that she will eventually give over to someone else. Even when she believes her motives are honorable, others will not always see it that way. The surrogate mother will be under considerable social pressure to break the agreement.

Surrogate mothers' motivations vary. Most surrogates are married and have already completed their families. Because many surrogates have had personal contact with infertility they believe they are doing a wonderful deed by giving the gift of life to an infertile couple. Others will admit they are doing it simply for the money.

Surrogate motherhood is risky and certainly the most controversial alternative for infertile couples. With the development of new technologies, there are fewer reasons today than in the past that prevent women from conceiving a child. Thus, before considering surrogacy, couples should carefully examine all other options to childbirth.

Child-Free Living

Couples who undergo several years of tests and treatment for infertility feel driven to succeed at pregnancy. They become involved in a power struggle with their bodies. As a result, succeeding at conception becomes the primary goal and clouds the previous motivations and desire for a child.

When infertility continues for many years, most couples need to step back and reexamine their motives for having a child. Some couples, as they are reevaluating their life goals, decide their desire to have a child has changed. They may realize, partially as a result of their infertility, that children are no guarantee of happiness and security. For others, options such as adoption or surrogacy will not be acceptable for them. These couples have come to the realization that they cannot give up their own pregnancy and nursing experience. Thus, some infertile couples will choose child-free living as an alternative to the already described options.

Living child-free should not be confused with living childless. The term childless implies settling for a life-style that was not really wanted. In contrast, child-free denotes a conscious, well-thought-out decision to stop being "infertile" and thus, to stop placing so much importance on "having" children.[23]

The idea of couples' consciously deciding not to have a child after putting so much time, effort, emotion, and money into having a child, may seem laughable. In fact, the child-free decision is not for everyone. Those who felt that their lives were empty were those who did not finish grieving for their unborn children. Those who have regretted their decision were those who did not enrich their lives in some way.[24] However, for many couples, the choice to remain child-free can be a very positive resolution to their infertility.

There are a few different types of child-free decisions that couples may consider. Some may practice contraception temporarily while they are trying to form a more permanent decision. Some couples may actively stop trying to conceive but would gladly welcome a pregnancy if Nature allowed it. For others, their resolution requires an act of closure in order to get on with their lives.[25] They need a definite conclusion to their battle with infertility and a commitment to their child-free decision. It can be a very difficult decision, but sterilization may be the answer. With sterilization there would be little room for second-guessing and no internal pressure about changing their decision.

The decision to remain child-free is often a lonely one. There may not be many people that couples can talk with about it. As parents will want to be grandparents and friends will want playmates for their children, couples may not find much support for their decision. Those friends who are parents may actually be offended, interpreting the child free decision as an affront on their life-style. Infertile friends may panic, thinking that they have not yet reached the inevitable decision to live child-free.

Couples' decision to remain child-free may also be misunderstood by others. Often it may be interpreted as selfish and self-centered. Despite studies that show that child-free couples are just as happy as those with children, many think that child-free couples cannot possibly be happy.[26] Regardless of what other people think, couples need to decide what is most important in life to them, and it does not necessarily have to be parenthood.

Couples who are successful at minimizing the desire for a biological child can proceed with choosing a life-style that is an alternative to parenting. Choosing a child-free life can open many doors to couples. Some may find themselves rekindling the relationship with their spouse that may have gotten lost during their bout with infertility. Other couples may use the time to continue their education, advance their careers, or simply develop new hobbies. For others, a life-long dream to travel now seems within reach.

The new-found energy that couples have after they have ended their struggle with infertility can be generated into many new areas. Some couples may find solace in volunteer work or may become involved with church activities. This new energy can also be channeled toward other people. Nieces and nephews may be seen in a new light for child-free couples. Becoming a Big Brother or Big Sister to an underprivileged child or offering to baby-sit for a friend's baby may be ways of satisfying that nurturing instinct. For many couples pets become an important part of their family.

> We've presented a very optimistic picture of what it means to be child-free. It was, for us, the happy ending to our infertility crises. After the silent fears of infertility had turned into certainty, after all hope of having children vanished, after the rage and despair and feelings of inadequacy, our lives are now better than they have ever been. We don't mean simply bearable or even as good as before. We mean better. Something good happened in the change from being infertile to being child-free.[27]

A Final Word to Counselors

When couples resolve their infertility, their lives take on a new positive focus. Their lives are no longer being controlled by their infertility. Instead, couples have a renewed purpose and direction. For those couples who achieve pregnancy, they prepare for their long-awaited child. For those who choose an alternate method to parenting: surrogacy, adoption, or AID, they also waiting for their child. However, they also have additional roadblocks to encounter. For those couples who choose a child-free life-style, they have a renewed sense of interest in pursuing their own happiness and self-fulfillment. For all groups, they give up their infertility to get on with living.

Although resolved couples have a decidedly more positive approach to life than before, they are not without problems. Self-doubt, second-guessing, and frustrations resulting from their infertility are expected. Counselors, clergy, and all helpers who are in contact with couples during this phase of their lives need to continue their encouragement and understanding. Couples need the encouragement to continue with their chosen lifestyle as well as the support and advice necessary to overcome the frustrations they will undoubtedly encounter.

Epilogue

We wrote this book during our son's first year of life. The joy we felt through that year enabled us to look back and relive some of the past hurts and problems. Because we were close enough to the hurts, they were still fresh in our minds. However, because of the emotional buffer provided by our son's presence in our lives, we were better able to understand intellectually the emotions from the experience.

Infertility continues to be a part of us, as we think about the possibility of another child. The anger returns as we think that our decision for a second child will be based as much on financial concerns—can we save the necessary money—as it will be on psychological readiness. However, the problem will not be impossible. We have been faced with more difficult problems and have grown. As a result of our infertility, we believe we can handle most anything life will throw at us.

We hope counselors find this book useful. We wanted to convey an understanding of the emotional issues confronted regularly by couples who face the challenge of infertility. Although all infertile couples may not seek counseling, all couples deal with emotions that are at times overwhelming. Couples who do seek help should be made aware of this, as they may find comfort in knowing that the emotions they are experiencing are expected and normal. Sections of this book may be used to reinforce this message, as we tried to provide real examples of how the emotions are confronted.

We tried to impart some basic knowledge about the medical aspects of infertility. Counselors, clergy, and other helpers can use this knowledge to feel better able to understand couples' medical experience. In addition, many of the references that are used through the book are from sources that can be given to couples. Many of these sources focus on the medical aspects of infertility and provide more detail about specific problems and procedures than we were able to give. Furthermore, as it is impossible to write about infertility without discussion of the emotional components, all the sources discuss the feelings couples experience as they cope with their infertility. Theses sources can provide additional validation for the couples' emotions.

Finally, to those counselors who find themselves working with couples or individuals who are infertile, we strongly recommend they learn about their local chapter of Resolve and about other local support groups for problems with infertility or pregnancy loss. These groups provide services that can be invaluable. In many cases, the feelings that are experienced by couples who are infertile can only be successfully addressed by others who are infertile. These groups will be especially helpful to couples who do not know other infertile couples.

Through this book, besides the knowledge acquired in our research and experience, we shared ourselves and our emotional confrontation with infertility. Others also shared with us so that they might be helpful to us and to others. Through this process, we learned that sharing helps. For us and others, sharing provides a purpose for the difficult experience. We are comforted in knowing that the difficulty we went through had some benefit. Thus, we hope this book will encourage couples who have suffered infertility and other pregnancy-related problems to share their experiences with others. They may be surprised by the outcome.

References

Chapter 1: A Woman's Perspective

1. R. Rhodes, "Women, Motherhood, and Infertility: The Social and Historical Context," *Infertility and Adoption: A Guide for Social Work Practice*, in ed., D. Valentine (New York: The Haworth Press, 1988), p. 11.
2. Ibid., p. 14.
3. Ibid., p. 16.
4. T. Seligson, "Success Isn't Enough: An Interview with Jamie Lee Curtis," *Parade Magazine* (October 29, 1989), p. 4–5.
5. K. Reed, M.N., "The Effect of Infertility on Female Sexuality," Pre- and Peri-Natal Psychology, vol. 2, 1 (Fall 1987), p. 58.
6. M. Sandelowski, R.N. and L. C. Jones, R. N. "Social Exchanges of Infertile Women," *Issues in Mental Health Nursing*, vol. 8 (1986), p. 175.
7. C. E. Miall, "The Stigma of Involuntary Childlessness," *Social Problems* 33, 4 (1984), p. 274.
8. B. E. Menning, "The Psychosocial Impact of Infertility," *Nursing Clinics of North America*, vol. 17, 1 (March 1982), p. 158.
9. V. J. Callan, "The Psychological Adjustment of Women Experiencing Infertility," *British Journal of Medical Psychology* 61, (1988), pp. 137–40.

Chapter 2: A Man's Perspective

1. D. Clements, "A Process of Understanding," *Resolve National Newsletter*, vol. 13, 5 (1988), p. 3.
2. M. H. Jones, "Beautiful Desire Led to This," Resolve reprint adapted from Resolve of Greater Hartford Conn. Newsletter (1984) Fall/Winter.
3. C. Harkness, *The Infertility Book; A Comprehensive Medical and Emotional Guide* (San Francisco: Volcano Press, Inc., 1987), p. 202.

4. E. Grima, "Mother's Day, Then Father's Day," Resolve reprint, adapted from Resolve of Michigan *Newsletter* June 1984.
5. D. Berger, "Couples' Reactions to Male Infertility and Donor Insemination," *American Journal of Psychiatry*, vol. 137, 9 (1980), pp. 1047–49.

Chapter 3: To Want a Child

1. K. Jensen, and editors of U.S. News Books, *Reproduction: The Cycle of Life* (Washington, D.C.: U.S. News and World Report, Inc., 1982), p. 17.
2. Ibid., pp. 9–10.
3. Ibid., p. 12.
4. Ibid., p. 13.
5. L. W. Hoffman and J. D. Manis, "The Value of Children in the United States: A New Approach to the Study of Fertility," *Journal of Marriage and the Family* (August 1979), p. 590.
6. L. N. Gupta, D. Srivastava, S. K. Verma, "Infertile Couples and Neuroticism," *Indian Journal of Clinical Psychology* 9 (1982), p. 64.
7. D. Entwisle. "Becoming a Parent," *The Handbook of Family Psychology and Therapy, Vol 1*, in ed. L. L'Abate, (Homewood, Illinois: Dorsey Press, 1985), p. 565.
8. C. E. Miall, "The Stigma of Involuntary Childlessness," *Social Problems* 33, 4 (1984), pp. 268–69.
9. J. W. Bardwick, "Evolution and Parenting," *Journal of Social Issues* 30, 4 (1974) pp. 39–62.
10. A. S. Rossi, "A Biosocial Perspective on Parenting," *Daedalus* 106 (1977), p. 2.
11. Boston Women's Health Book Collective, *Our Bodies, Ourselves* (New York: Simon and Schuster, 1976), p. 246.
12. R. Kastenbaum, "Fertility and the Fear of Death," *Journal of Social Issues* 30, 4 (1974) p. 64.
13. P. Aries, *Centuries of Childhood* (New York: Knopf, 1962), p. 36.
14. S. Freud, "On Narcissism: An Introduction," *Collected Papers of Sigmund Freud, vol. 4*, (London: Hogarth Press, 1953) (Originally Published in 1914).
15. Ibid.
16. L. W. Hoffman and J. D. Manis, "The Value of Children in the United States: A New Approach to the Study of Fertility," *Journal of Marriage and the Family* (August 1979), p. 585.
17. Ibid.
18. L. W. Hoffman and F. Wyatt, "Social Change and Motivation for Having Larger Families: Some Theoretical Considerations," in ed.

J. Edwards, *The Family and Social Change* (New York: Knopf, 1969), p. 178.

19. L. W. Hoffman and J. D. Manis, "The Value of Children in the United States: A New Approach to the Study of Fertility," *Journal of Marriage and the Family* (August, 1979) p. 588.

20. L. Braverman, "The Myth of Motherhood," *Women in Families: A Framework for Family Therapy.* in ed. M. McGoldrick, C. Anderson, and F. Walsh (New York: Norton and Co., 1989), p. 228.

21. J. J. Stangel, *The New Fertility and Conception: The Essential Guide for Childless Couples* (New York and Scarborough, Ontario: New American Library, 1988), p. 4.

22. S. J. Silber, *How to Get Pregnant* (New York: Warner Books, 1980), p. 11.

23. J. J. Stangel, *The New Fertility and Conception; The Essential Guide for Childless Couples* (New York and Scarborough, Ontario: New American Library, 1988), p. 217.

24. Ibid., p. 6.

Chapter 4: Beginning the Struggle with Infertility

1. J. J. Stangel, *The New Fertility and Conception: The Essential Guide for Childless Couples*, p. 6.

2. N. Lauersen and E. Stukane, *Listen to Your Body: A Gynecologist Answers Women's Most Intimate Questions* (New York: Berkley Books, 1983), p. 178.

3. Ibid., pp. 178–79.

4. C. E. Miall, "The Stigma of Involuntary Childlessness," *Social Problems* 33, 4 (1984): p. 269.

5. M. J. Frisch and G. Rapoport, *Getting Pregnant!* (Tucson, Arizona: The Body Press, 1987), p. 4.

6. C. Harkness, *The Infertility Book; A Comprehensive Medical and Emotional Guide*, pp. 117, 135, 145, 149, 152.

7. Ibid., p. 128.

8. B. E. Menning, *Infertility; A Guide for the Childless Couple* (New York: Prentice-Hall Press, 1977), p. 44.

9. C. Harkness, *The Infertility Book; A Comprehensive Medical and Emotional Guide*, p. 193.

10. Ibid., p. 189.

11. Ibid., p. 195.

12. Ibid., pp. 195–96.

13. Ibid., p. 196.

14. K. L. McEwan, C. G. Costello, and P. J. Taylor, "Adjustment to Infertility," *Journal of Abnormal Psychology* 96, 2 (1987), p. 108.

15. B. E. Menning, *Infertility; A Guide for the Childless Couple*, pp. 110–22.

16. A. Hill, "Infertility as Posttraumatic Stress Disorder," Resolve *National Newsletter* 14, 2 (1989), p. 8.

17. J. Fleming, "Infertility as a Chronic Illness," Resolve *National Newsletter* (December 1984).

18. M. Sandelowski, "The Color Gray: Ambiguity and Infertility," *IMAGE: Journal of Nursing Scholarship*, vol. 19, 2 and (Summer 1987), pp. 70–74.

19. J. Hudson and S. Danish, "The Acquisition of Information: An Important Life Skill," *The Personnel and Guidance Journal*, 59, 3 (1980), pp. 164–67.

Chapter 5: Advanced Infertility

1. D. Clapp, "What Is an Infertility Specialist?: (And How To Get the Best Medical Care)," reprinted from the Resolve *National Newsletter*, (June, 1987).

2. L. M. Wallace, "Psychological Adjustment to and Recovery from Laparoscopic Sterilization and Infertility Investigation," *Journal of Psychosomatic Research*, vol. 29, 5 (1985), p. 517.

3. M. J. Frisch and G. Rapoport, *Getting Pregnant!* (Tucson, Arizona: The Body Press, 1987), p. 165.

4. C. Harkness, *The Infertility Book; A Comprehensive Medical and Emotional Guide*, p. 146.

5. K. Schwan, *The Infertility Maze; Finding Your Way to the Right Help and the Right Answers*, (Chicago: Contemporary Books, 1988), p. 156.

6. J. J. Stangel, *The New Fertility and Conception; The Essential Guide for Childless Couples*, p. 113.

7. B. E. Menning, *Infertility; A Guide for the Childless Couple*, p. 84.

8. K. Schwan, *The Infertility Maze; Finding Your Way to the Right Help and the Right Answers*, p. 185.

9. Ibid., pp. 190–91.

10. S. K. Needleman, "Infertility and In-Vitro Fertilization: The Social Worker's Role," *Health and Social Work* (Spring 1987), p. 140.

11. D. A. Greenfield, M. P. Diamond, and A. H. DeCherney, "Grief Reactions Following In-Vitro Fertilization Treatment," *Journal of Psychosomatic Obstetrics and Gynaecology* 8 (1988), p. 170.

12. L. Salzer, "The Emotional Experience of IVF," Resolve *National Newsletter*, vol. 13, 5 (December 1988), p. 5.

13. D. A. Greenfield, M. P. Diamond, and A. H. DeCherney, "Grief Reactions Following In-Vitro Fertilization Treatment," *Journal of Psychosomatic Obstetrics and Gynaecology* 8 (1988), pp. 170–71.

14. H. Seyle, *The Stress of Life* (New York: McGraw-Hill, 1978); p. 159–168.

15. M. Sandelowski. "The Color Gray: Ambiguity and Infertility," *Image: Journal of Nursing Scholarship*, vol. 19, 2 (Summer 1987), pp. 70–74.

16. B. E. Menning, *Infertility; A Guide for the Childless Couple*, pp. 119–22.

17. A. Ellis, *Reason and Emotion in Psychotherapy* (New York: Lyle Stuart Press, 1962).

18. D. Meichenbaum, *Cognitive-Behavior Modification* (New York: Plenum Press, 1977).

19. I. Yalom, *The Theory and Practice of Group Psychotherapy* (New York: Basic Books, 1975), pp. 3–18.

Chapter 6: Marital Issues

1. M. Korda, "If You Look to Marriage as an Instrument for Personal Growth," in *Marriage Today: Problems, Issues and Alternatives*, ed. J. E. DeBerger (New York: Wiley and Sons, 1977), p. 664.

2. L. W. Hoffman and J. D. Manis, "The Value of Children in the United States: A New Approach to the Study of Fertility," *Journal of Marriage and the Family* (August 1979), p. 588.

3. D. M. Berger, "Couples' Reactions to Male Infertility and Donor Insemination," *American Journal of Psychiatry*, vol. 137, 9 (September 1980), p. 1048.

4. D. Sahaj, K. Smith, K. Kimmel, R. Houesknecht, R. Hewes, B. Meyer, L. Leduc, and A. Danford, "A Psychosocial Description of a Select Group of Infertile Couples," *The Journal of Family Practice*, vol. 27, 4 (1988), pp. 393–97.

5. B. E. Menning, *Infertility; A Guide for the Childless Couple*, pp. 110–22.

6. J. C. Daniluk, A Leader, and P. Taylor. "Psychological and Relationship Changes of Couples Undergoing an Infertility Investigation: Some Implications for Counsellors," *British Journal of Guidance and Counseling*, vol. 15, 1 (January 1987), pp. 29–36.

7. D. Powell, *Understanding Human Adjustment* (Boston: Little, Brown and Associates, 1983), p. 75.

8. J. Gottman, C. Notarius, J. Gonso, and H. Markman, *A Couple's Guide to Communication* (Champaign, Ill.: Research Press, 1976), p. 1.

9. Ibid., pp. 47–48.

Chapter 7: Loss

1. B. E. Menning, *Infertility; A Guide for the Childless Couple*, p. 116.
2. Ibid., p. 118.
3. J. Bowlby, *Attachment and Loss, vol. 3, Loss: Sadness and Depression* (New York: Basic Books Inc., 1980), p. 85.
4. B. E. Menning, *Infertility; A Guide for the Childless Couple*, p. 111–13.
5. S. Semchyshyn and C. Colman, *How to Prevent Miscarriage and Other Crises of Pregnancy* (New York: Macmillan Publishing Company, 1989), p. 22.
6. B. E. Menning, *Infertility; A Guide for the Childless Couple*, p. 69.
7. C. Harkness, *The Infertility Book; A Comprehensive Medical and Emotional Guide*, p. 154.
8. N. A. Bowers, "Early Pregnancy Loss in the Infertile Couple," *Journal of Obstetrics and Gynecologic Neonatal Nursing* (JOGNN) (Supplement) (November/December 1985), p. 56s.
9. S. Semchyshyn and C. Colman, *How to Prevent Miscarriage and Other Crises of Pregnancy*, p. 17.
10. Ibid., p. 56.
11. C. Harkness, *The Infertility Book; A Comprehensive Medical and Emotional Guide*, p. 155.
12. M. Beck, M. Hager, I. Wickelgren, L. Brown, D. Foote, and L. Wright, "Miscarriages," *Newsweek* (August 15, 1988), p. 47.
13. L. Plouffe, Jr. and P. G. McDonough, "Multiple Miscarriage," Resolve reprint (January 1989).
14. S. Semchyshyn and C. Colman, *How to Prevent Miscarriage and Other Crises of Pregnancy*, p. 2.
15. Ibid., p. 15.
16. Ibid., p. 207.
17. J. J. Stangel, *The New Fertility and Conception: The Essential Guide for Childless Couples*, p. 145–46.
18. M. Beck, M. Hager, I. Wickelgren, L. Brown, D. Foote, and L. Wright, "Miscarriages," p. 46.
19. C. Harkness, *The Infertility Book; A Comprehensive Medical and Emotional Guide*, p. 163.
20. S. Semchyshyn and C. Colman, *How to Prevent Miscarriage and Other Crises of Pregnancy*, p. 71.
21. B. E. Menning, *Infertility; A Guide for the Childless Couple*, p. 80.
22. C. Harkness, *The Infertility Book; A Comprehensive Medical and Emotional Guide*, p. 165.
23. C. C. Floyd, "Pregnancy After Reproductive Failure," *American Journal of Nursing* (November 1981), p. 2051.

Chapter 8: Resolved

1. B. E. Menning, *Infertility; A Guide for the Childless Couple*, p. 119.
2. D. Clapp, "Emotional Responses to Infertility: Nursing Interventions," *Journal of Obstetrics and Gynecologic Neonatal Nursing* (JOGNN) (Supplement), (November/December 1985), p. 34s.
3. B. E. Menning, *Infertility; A Guide for the Childless Couple*, pp. 119–20.
4. C. H. Garner, "Pregnancy After Infertility," *Journal of Obstetrics and Gynecologic Neonatal Nursing* (JOGNN) (Supplement), (November/December 1985), p. 59s.
5. M. Humphrey, *The Hostage Seekers: A Study of Childless and Adopting Couples* (United Kingdom: Longmans, 1969).
6. N. Gibbs, "The Baby Chase," *Time* (October 9, 1989), p. 86.
7. H. Kirk, *Adoptive Kinship: A Modern Institution in Need of Reform* (Toronto: Butterworths, 1981).
8. C. E. Miall, "The Stigma of Adoptive Parent Status: Perceptions of Community Attitudes Toward Adoption and the Experience of Informal Social Sanctioning," *Family Relations* (January 1987), pp. 34–39.
9. Ibid., pp. 34–39.
10. Ibid., pp. 34–39.
11. M. Ward, "Parental Bonding in Older Child Adoption," *Child Welfare* 60 (1981), p. 25.
12. A. Baran, R. Pannor, and A. Sorosky, "Adoptive Parents and the Sealed Record Controversy," *Social Casework* (1974), pp. 531–36.
13. C. E. Miall, "The Stigma of Adoptive Parent Status: Perceptions of Community Attitudes Toward Adoption and the Experience of Informal Social Sanctioning," *Family Relations* (January 1987), p. 36.
14. D. W. LaPere, "Vulnerability to Crises During the Life Cycle of the Adoptive Family," in *Infertility and Adoption: A Guide for Social Work Practice*, ed. D. Valentine, (New York: The Haworth Press, 1988), p. 80–82.
15. C. Harkness, *The Infertility Book; A Comprehensive Medical and Emotional Guide*, p. 220.
16. N. Gibbs, "The Baby Chase," *Time* (October 9, 1989), p. 86.
17. C. Harkness, *The Infertility Book; A Comprehensive Medical and Emotional Guide*, p. 204.
18. Ibid., p. 209.
19. Ibid., p. 208.
20. Ibid., p. 206.
21. D. M. Berger, "Couples' Reactions to Male Infertility and Donor

Insemination," *American Journal of Psychiatry*, vol. 137, 9 (September 1980), p. 1048.

22. C. Harkness, *The Infertility Book; A Comprehensive Medical and Emotional Guide*, p. 205.

23. J. W. Carter and M. Carter, *Sweet Grapes: How to Stop Being Infertile and Start Living Again* (Indianapolis, Indiana: Perspective Press, 1989), pp. 13–15.

24. M. Bombardieri, "Childfree Decision-Making," Reprint from Resolve Inc. 1989, p. 2.

25. J. W. Carter and M. Carter, *Sweet Grapes: How to Stop Being Infertile and Start Living Again*, p. 71.

26. M. Bombardieri, "Childfree Decision-Making," p. 4.

27. J. W. Carter and M. Carter, *Sweet Grapes: How to Stop Being Infertile and Start Living Again*, p. 41.

THE CONTINUUM
COUNSELING LIBRARY
Books of Related Interest

_____Denyse Beaudet
ENCOUNTERING THE MONSTER
Pathways in Children's Dreams
Based on original empirical research, and with recourse to the
works of Jung, Neumann, Eliade, Marie-Louise Franz, and
others, this book offers proven methods of approaching and
understanding the dream life of children. $17.95

_____Robert W. Buckingham
CARE OF THE DYING CHILD
A Practical Guide for Those Who Help Others
"Buckingham's book delivers a powerful, poignant message
deserving a wide readership."—*Library Journal* $17.95

_____Alastair V. Campbell, ed.
A DICTIONARY OF PASTORAL CARE
Provides information on the essentials of counseling and the
kinds of problems encountered in pastoral practice. The approach is interdenominational and interdisciplinary. Contains
over 300 entries by 185 authors in the fields of theology, philoso-
phy, psychology, and sociology as well as from the theoretical
background of psychotherapy and counseling. $24.50

_____David A. Crenshaw
BEREAVEMENT
Counseling the Grieving throughout the Life Cycle
Grief is examined from a life cycle perspective, infancy to old
age. Special losses and practical strategies for frontline
caregivers highlight this comprehensive guidebook. $16.95

_____Reuben Fine
THE HISTORY OF PSYCHOANALYSIS
New Expanded Edition
"Objective, comprehensive, and readable. A rare work. Highly
recommended, whether as an introduction to the field or as a
fresh overview to those already familiar with it."—*Contemporary
Psychology* $24.95 paperback

_____Reuben Fine
LOVE AND WORK
The Value System of Psychoanalysis
One of the world's leading authorities on Freud sheds new light
on psychoanalysis as a process for releasing the power of love.
$24.95

_____Raymond B. Flannery, Jr.
BECOMING STRESS-RESISTANT
Through the Project SMART Program
"An eminently practical book with the goals of helping men and
women of the 1990s make changes in their lives."—Charles V.
Ford, Academy of Psychosomatic Medicine $17.95

_____Lucy Freeman
FIGHT AGAINST FEARS
With a new Introduction by
Flora Rheta Schreiber
More than a million copies sold. The new—and only available—
edition of the first, and still best, true story of a modern woman's
journey of self-discovery through psychoanalysis.
$10.95 paperback

_____Lucy Freeman
OUR INNER WORLD OF RAGE
Understanding and Transforming the Power of Anger
A psychoanalytic examination of the anger that burns within us
and which can be used to save or slowly destroy us. Sheds light
on all expressions of rage, from the murderer to the suicide to
those of us who feel depressed and angry but are unaware of the
real cause. $9.95 paperback

_____ John Gerdtz and Joel Bregman, M. D.
AUTISM
A Practical Guide for Those Who Help Others
An up-to-date and comprehensive guidebook for everyone who works with autistic children, adolescents, adults, and their families. Includes latest information on medications. $17.95

_____Marion Howard
**HOW TO HELP YOUR TEENAGER
POSTPONE SEXUAL INVOLVEMENT**
Based on a national educational program that works, this book advises parents, teachers, and counselors on how they can help their teens resist social and peer pressures regarding sex.
$9.95 paperback

_____Marion Howard
SOMETIMES I WONDER ABOUT ME
Teenagers and Mental Health
Combines fictional narratives with sound, understandable professional advice to help teenagers recognize the difference between serious problems and normal problems of adjustment.
$9.95

_____Charles H. Huber and Barbara A. Backlund
THE TWENTY MINUTE COUNSELOR
Transforming Brief Conversations into Effective
Helping Experiences
Expert advice for anyone who by necessity must often counsel "on the run" or in a short period of time. $16.95

_____E. Clay Jorgensen
CHILD ABUSE
A Practical Guide for Those Who Help Others
Essential information and practical advice for caregivers called upon to help both child and parent in child abuse. $16.95

_____Eugene Kennedy
CRISIS COUNSELING
The Essential Guide for Nonprofessional Counselors
"An outstanding author of books on personal growth selects
types of personal crises that our present life-style has made
commonplace and suggests effective ways to deal with them."
—*Best Sellers* $10.95

_____Eugene Kennedy and Sara Charles, M. D.
ON BECOMING A COUNSELOR
A Basic Guide for Nonprofessional Counselors
New expanded edition of an indispensable resource. A patient-
oriented, clinically directed field guide to understanding and
responding to troubled people. $27.95 hardcover
$15.95 paperback

_____Eugene Kennedy
SEXUAL COUNSELING
A Practical Guide for Those Who Help Others
Newly revised and up-to-date edition, with a new chapter on
the counselor and AIDS, of an essential book on counseling
people with sexual problems. $17.95

_____Bonnie Lester
WOMEN AND AIDS
A Practical Guide for Those Who Help Others
Provides positive ways for women to deal with their fears, and
to help others who react with fear to people who have AIDS.
$15.95

_____Robert J. Lovinger
RELIGION AND COUNSELING
The Psychological Impact of Religious Belief
How counselors and clergy can best understand the important
emotional significance of religious thoughts and feelings. $17.95

_____Helen B. McDonald and Audrey I. Steinhorn
HOMOSEXUALITY
A Practical Guide to Counseling Lesbians, Gay Men, and Their Families
A sensitive guide to better understanding and counseling gays, lesbians, and their parents, at every stage of their lives. $17.95

_____ James McGuirk and Mary Elizabeth McGuirk
FOR WANT OF A CHILD
A Psychologist and His Wife Explore the Emotional Effects and Challenges of Infertility
A new understanding of infertility that comes from one couple's lived experience, as well as sound professional advice for couples and counselors. $17.95

_____ Janice N. McLean and Sheila A. Knights
PHOBICS AND OTHER PANIC VICTIMS
A Practical Guide for Those Who Help Them
"A must for the phobic, spouse and family, and for the physician and support people who help them. It can spell the difference between partial therapy with partial results and comprehensive therapy and recovery." — Arthur B. Hardy, M. D., Founder, TERRAP Phobia Program $15.95

_____ John B. Mordock and William Van Ornum
CRISIS COUNSELING WITH CHILDREN AND ADOLESCENTS
A Guide for Nonprofessional Counselors
New Expanded Edition
"Every parent should keep this book on the shelf right next to the nutrition, medical, and Dr. Spock books."—*Marriage & Family Living* $12.95

_____ John B. Mordock
COUNSELING CHILDREN
Basic Principles for Helping the Troubled and Defiant Child
Helps counselors consider the best route for a particular child,
and offers proven principles and methods to counsel troubled
children in a variety of situations. $17.95

_____Cherry Boone O'Neill
DEAR CHERRY
Questions and Answers on Eating Disorders
Practical and inspiring advice on eating disorders from the best-
selling author of *Starving for Attention.* $8.95

_____Paul G. Quinnett
**ON BECOMING A HEALTH
AND HUMAN SERVICES MANAGER**
A Practical Guide for Clinicians and Counselors
A new and essential guide to management for everyone in the
helping professions—from mental health to nursing, from social
work to teaching. $19.95

_____Paul G. Quinnett
SUICIDE: THE FOREVER DECISION
For Those Thinking About Suicide,
and For Those Who Know, Love, or Counsel Them
"A treasure— this book can help save lives. It will be especially
valuable not only to those who are thinking about suicide but to
such nonprofessional counselors as teachers, clergy, doctors,
nurses, and to experienced therapists."—William Van Ornum,
psychotherapist and author $18.95 hardcover $8.95 paperback

_____Paul G. Quinnett
WHEN SELF-HELP FAILS
A Consumer's Guide to Counseling Services
A guide to professional therapie. "Without a doubt one of the
most honest, reassuring, nonpaternalistic, and useful self-help
books ever to appear."—*Booklist* $10.95

_____Judah L. Ronch
ALZHEIMER'S DISEASE
A Practical Guide for Those Who Help Others
Must reading for everyone who must deal with the effects of this
tragic disease on a daily basis. Filled with examples as well as
facts, this book provides insights into dealing with one's feelings
as well as with such practical advice as how to choose long-term
care. $11.95 paperback

_____Theodore Isaac Rubin, M. D.
ANTI-SEMITISM : A DISEASE OF THE MIND
"A most poignant and lucid psychological examination of a
severe emotional disease. Dr. Rubin offers hope and under-
standing to the victim and to the bigot. A splendid job!"
—Dr. Herbert S. Strean $14.95

_____Theodore Isaac Rubin, M.D.
CHILD POTENTIAL
Fulfilling Your Child's Intellectual, Emotional, and Creative Promise
Information, guidance, and wisdom—a treasury of fresh ideas
for parents to help their children become their best selves
without professional help. $17.95

_____John R. Shack
COUPLES COUNSELING
A Practical Guide for Those Who Help Others
An essential guide to dealing with the 20 percent of all counsel-
ing situations that involve the relationship of two people. $17.95

_____Stuart Sutherland
THE INTERNATIONAL DICTIONARY OF PSYCHOLOGY
This new dictionary of psychology also covers a wide range of
related disciplines, from anthropology to sociology. $49.95

_____ Joan Leslie Taylor
IN THE LIGHT OF DYING
The Journals of a Hospice Volunteer
A rare and beautiful book about death and dying that affirms life
and will inspire an attitude of love. "Beautifully recounts the
healing (our own) that results from service to others, and might
well be considered as required reading for hospice volunteers."
—Stephen Levine, author of *Who Dies?* $17.95

_____ Montague Ullman, M. D. and Claire Limmer, M. S., eds.
THE VARIETY OF DREAM EXPERIENCE
Expanding Our Ways of Working With Dreams
"Lucidly describes the beneficial impact dream analysis can have
in diverse fields and in society as a whole. An erudite, illuminat-
ing investigation."—*Booklist*
$19.95 hardcover $14.95 paperback

_____ William Van Ornum and Mary W. Van Ornum
TALKING TO CHILDREN ABOUT NUCLEAR WAR
"A wise book. A needed book. An urgent book."
—Dr. Karl A. Menninger $15.95 hardcover $7.95 paperback

_____ Kathleen Zraly and David Swift, M. D.
ANOREXIA, BULIMIA, AND COMPULSIVE OVEREATING
A Practical Guide for Counselors and Families
A psychiatrist and an eating disorders specialist provide new
and helpful approaches for everyone who knows, loves, or
counsels victims of anorexia, bulimia, and chronic overeating.
$17.95

At your bookstore, or to order directly, send your check or
money order (adding $2.00 extra per book for postage and
handling, up to $6.00 maximum) to: The Continuum Publishing
Company, 370 Lexington Avenue, New York, NY , 10017. Prices
are subject to change.